THE DeMARCO FACTOR

DATE DUE

D0972753

THE
DeMARCO
FACTOR

Transforming Public Will into Political Power

Michael Pertschuk

Vanderbilt University Press ■ Nashville

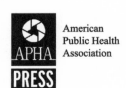

American
Public Health
Association

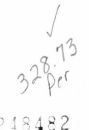

© 2010 by Michael Pertschuk
Published by Vanderbilt University Press
Nashville, Tennessee 37235
First printing 2010
Second printing 2010

This book is printed on acid-free paper
made from 30% post-consumer recycled content.
Manufactured in the United States of America

Library of Congress Cataloging-in-Publication Data
Pertschuk, Michael, 1933–
The DeMarco factor : transforming public will into
political power / Michael Pertschuk.
p. cm.
Includes index.
ISBN 978-0-8265-1702-9 (cloth : alk. paper)
ISBN 978-0-8265-1703-6 (pbk. : alk. paper)
1. Lobbying—United States—Case studies. 2. Public interest—United States—
Case studies. 3. DeMarco, Vincent. 4. Lobbyists—Maryland. 5. Antismoking
movement—Maryland. 6. Tobacco industry—Government policy—Maryland.
7. Antismoking movement—United States. 8. Tobacco industry—Government
policy—United States. I. Title.
JK1118.P46 2010
328.73′078—dc22
2009026820

Without the concentrating effort of a ... campaign, [political passion] dissipated into an attitude rather than any concrete program, a collection of grievances and not an organized force, images and sounds that crowd the airways and conversation but without any corporeal existence.

—Barack Obama, *Dreams from My Father*

For Anna

Contents

Introduction

I first learned of Vincent "Vinny" DeMarco in 1993. I was at the
Advocacy Institute in Washington, D.C., helping to train a new generation of
public health and social justice advocates. We were not immodest about some
of our achievements, especially our efforts to help build an effective national
tobacco control movement. Then an old colleague and good friend visited us
and issued a challenge: "Tobacco control is nice. Now try something hard.
Figure out how to get something done about controlling handguns."

In 1993, all I knew about gun control in the United States was that it was a
godforsaken cause. For years, the National Rifle Association (NRA) had systematically shuffled off into political oblivion any politician with the temerity
to challenge the association by proposing even the most modest constraints
on personal armories. Partly rising to our friend's dare—and partly because
she offered us an enticing grant from the foundation she ran—we agreed to
undertake a survey of gun control campaigns around the country, looking for
signs of life. We read everything we could find about gun control advocacy
efforts. We convened from around the country people who were active and
knowledgeable in such efforts, and we sought to learn who among all those
working to control guns was making significant progress. At the end of a
year of inquiry (and of the grant), we realized that all roads led next door to
Maryland.

In that state, we learned, a strong, diverse coalition had emerged: Marylanders Against Handgun Abuse. There had been not one, but a series of successful, innovative campaigns to cut down the profusion of lethal handguns,
especially in the state's inner cities. And behind the group was a community
organizer and strategist, Vincent DeMarco. I made it my business to meet this
DeMarco. As we talked, I learned that in his campaigns he had ignored much
of what we and others had learned and taught over the years about citizen
advocacy. Instead, he had developed his own methods for organizing and mo-

bilizing public support into a formidable political force capable of challenging even the NRA, that most potent lobby.

Soon we invited DeMarco to help us at the Advocacy Institute train aspiring advocates, not just in gun control, but also in other policy arenas facing formidable economic and political opposition. Since then, I have observed in awe and fascination—and with no little professional envy—as he has embarked on a series of advocacy campaigns, building each on the foundations and lessons of the preceding effort, as he has become what one journalist, not without respect, called Maryland's "serial campaigner."

By 1996, DeMarco had defeated the NRA in intense legislative combat in the Maryland General Assembly and in a statewide referendum. In 1997, he was recruited into tobacco control advocacy by a frustrated state coalition, and he proceeded to defeat Big Tobacco by persuading and pressuring the Maryland legislature—until then immobilized by the mythically formidable tobacco lobby—to mandate a significant leap in the state's tobacco tax. At that time I started to think about writing a book about DeMarco, his innovative strategies, and the nature of his leadership.

By 1999, he had embarked on yet another venture: to bring "health care for all" to Maryland. By 2004, he had begun to achieve a series of significant, if modest, steps toward that ambitious goal. With a book now seriously in mind, I began a series of taped interviews with him.

By 2006, DeMarco had defeated Wal-Mart's media propagandists and the corporation's lobbyists in the Maryland legislature by achieving the enactment of the only state law mandating that Wal-Mart raise the proportion of its payroll dedicated to health care for its workers—in the process overturning a veto by a governor in thrall to corporate interests. The law spurred the introduction of copycat bills in more than thirty states, a national momentum thwarted only by a federal court decision holding the law invalid—in conflict with federal law.

As this book was approaching its end in the spring of 2009, DeMarco had built Faith United Against Tobacco, an all-embracing national coalition of faith groups, from the peace-loving Methodists to the abortion-loathing Southern Baptists, enabling the Campaign for Tobacco-Free Kids to secure overwhelming bipartisan congressional passage of its long-sought federal goal: broad and powerful control by the U.S. Food and Drug Administration (FDA) of every element of cigarette manufacturing and marketing.

And now, a tantalizing possibility: as the book's narrative ends in the spring of 2009, the United States is led by a president who, like DeMarco, is an experienced community organizer, a president who speaks in terms of "we," not "I," as the potential counterforce to the corporate and other special interest lobbies that have dominated the national policy agenda for far too long. Although the new administration of Barack Obama has already accomplished much, some key elements of his program appear threatened by those same forces of reaction and political partisanship. For the 2010 congressional elections and beyond, DeMarco's unique breadth of organizing and his focus on election campaigns as vehicles for extracting pledges from legislators, who otherwise face voter revolt, may offer a model that could help our organizer president (and others after him) achieve the vision for change that helped get him elected.

The Organization of This Book

Parts I, II, and III of this book are campaign stories. In Part I, I narrate the ups and downs of the DeMarco-led 1997–1998 cigarette tax campaign, the Maryland Children's Initiative. I also draw portraits of DeMarco's history and his core team in action. But, like any story from life, it's selective. It dwells on those aspects of the campaign that highlight DeMarco's unique strategic template, marching in as orderly a fashion as political action allows through the entire campaign, some six discrete stages, each with its tailored campaign strategies and tactics—a model campaign. From time to time, I highlight the noteworthy strategic or tactical significance of actions taken and the potentially replicable nature of DeMarco's leadership qualities.

Part II, which focuses on DeMarco's 1999–2008 Maryland Health Care for All! campaign, is a more truncated narrative. Unlike the comparatively seamless cigarette tax campaign, this "chameleon campaign" underwent many abrupt changes in the course of a series of incremental subcampaigns. While further illuminating DeMarco's basic strategies, in this part of the book I focus on his ability to develop, and continuously adapt, coherent campaign strategies for a highly complex goal; his response to unanticipated political disasters; his ability to sustain a broad-based and energetic coalition for nearly ten years; and, without compromising goals or principles, his flexibility in accommodating the needs and desires of the essential inside leaders—the governors, house speakers, senate presidents, and key committee chairs.

The activities that make up Part III, which tracks DeMarco's work with the national Campaign for Tobacco-Free Kids, include what, for me, were the biggest surprises. I had not foreseen that in the process of researching this work, I would unearth new dimensions in DeMarco's contributions to advocacy support, an enrichment of his strategies on a national scale, and above all revelations about the power and effect of the grand alliances he forges between the health advocacy and faith communities. I also discovered the synergistic energy generated when DeMarco joins forces with that rare occurrence: a public interest advocacy organization that is deep in both human expertise and financial resources.

Advocacy Strategic and Leadership Lessons

Part IV moves away from the campaign stories and is directed especially toward advocates and students of advocacy. Toward the end of my tenure at the Advocacy Institute, DeMarco presented case studies of his campaigns that proved eye opening and popular. To draw lessons from such case studies, we and our students tested them against a deceptively simple but proven method of strategic planning for policy advocacy campaigns: the Nine Questions, developed by our colleague Jim Shultz, executive director of the Democracy Center (formerly Advocacy Institute West).

At the Advocacy Institute, David Cohen, Kathleen Sheekey, and I also developed—and have continuously tinkered with—what we call a Leadership Taxonomy to help convey to our trainees the essence of successful issue advocacy leadership. We found that successful campaigns seemed to require a complement of individuals who could fill several distinct roles. Our taxonomy identified and sought to capture the qualities essential to each. At the institute, the taxonomy proved useful in training coalition leaders and other advocates to scan and assess the complement of leaders they were working with, as well as their own leadership roles—to identify, and then seek to fill their leadership gaps.

The introduction to Part IV includes a description of Shultz's Nine Question strategic planning process. My analysis of where and how DeMarco's campaign templates, strategies, and tactics fit within the Nine Question framework makes up Chapters 13 and 14. In Chapter 15, I present the Leadership Taxonomy, locate within it DeMarco's strengths and limits, and ask which leadership roles DeMarco inhabits and how well he manages to compensate for those leadership qualities he does not himself possess.

Methodology

This is not an arms-length book. I am not, with respect to DeMarco—as someone once observed about my public work—"a neutral noodle," so I want to be transparent about the methodology of this book. I have written it because I greatly respect Vincent DeMarco's leadership and strategies. Over more than fifteen years, he has become a good friend and colleague, and nothing I discovered through the deeper investigation of his work for this book disillusioned me. To the contrary, I learned much about his work and many lessons from him that I had not understood well before.

With respect to DeMarco and his colleagues, I relied heavily on the transcripts of extensive interviews I conducted with those who worked with him and closely observed him, with these ground rules:

The interviews were recorded and subsequently transcribed.

I excerpted them, in the process pruning verbal stumbles and repetition. I moved phrases and sentences around for clarity and flow. In places, I asked for clarification or expansion from the interviewee. But in all cases, the words quoted are those of the person interviewed.

To gain the interviewees' complete comfort and candor, I promised each the opportunity to review what I had excerpted in the context of draft chapters of this book.

I encouraged each interviewee to make factual corrections, raise questions, complain, and urge changes of text that might cause pain to others or to suggest where I was missing the heart of the story or being unfair.

People interviewed had no veto power, just the opportunity to plead (even whine). I discouraged any plea for revision simply to polish the natural flow of the spoken word because I wanted very much to capture the authentic voices of those interviewed—how the key players thought and spoke to each other when no stranger was listening.

No one sought to abuse these ground rules. DeMarco himself never complained about being placed in an unfair light; instead, he reserved his plea bargaining for places where he felt I had unfairly treated others. We worked out these concerns to our mutual satisfaction.

I reached out to some of DeMarco's critics and pressed his allies for his flaws and foibles. Some of the most telling criticisms came from his fondest coworkers, until, that is, I interviewed the strongest of his opponents in many of the campaigns documented herein—veteran state tobacco industry lobbyist Bruce Bereano. Bereano scorns and loathes DeMarco and, though I cannot agree with his arguments and judgments, I present them faithfully throughout. I am indeed grateful to Bereano, a colleague when I was a staff member working in the U.S. Senate during the 1970s, for his willingness to be interviewed and to speak with candor and passion at length, and on the record.

Though I owe much gratitude to many who more than helped me wend my way through the narratives and analyses in this book (see the acknowledgments), one exceptional gift needs to be acknowledged here. As I researched the book and scoured the pages of the *Baltimore Sun* for facts and details of the DeMarco campaigns, C. Fraser Smith, long the *Sun's* senior political analyst and commentator, kept surfacing as a singular voice wryly observing DeMarco's progress and stumbles. I could not hope to match Smith's canny insights into Maryland politics, his eloquence and wit, or his appreciation for DeMarco's role. It is from one of his columns that I have filched the book's title. But far more, I have used his timely words not sparingly throughout, as a one-person Greek chorus, giving light and insight to the DeMarco factor.

Vincent DeMarco is making an important contribution to the avowed democratic promise of transforming public will into public policy. All of us who seek to help make that promise reality can learn much from him, and that is why I wrote this book. DeMarco is also a colorful, delightful, if sometimes maddening human being, as this book reflects. As a prelude, I offer this perceptively balanced recollection from DeMarco's close colleague and friend, Baltimore bishop Douglas Miles, as he relates their first meeting:

> I thought, Who is this guy? He does not strike you as a lobbyist. He does not strike you as a super professional. In fact, he showed up at the interview with his boy on his arm and wrestled with his boy the whole time that he was talking with me. Of course, a kid doesn't want to sit through a meeting with adults with nothing to do. And I'm sitting there saying, Who is this guy?
>
> He looks like Columbo [the deceptively disheveled and bumbling TV detective]. It's kind of a persona, but his is not a put-on, not an act that he was using to throw people off. What you see is what you get. I've never met a more authentic person. There is no pretense; there is no put-on with Vinny. He's an extraordinarily committed person, a very bright person, and one who knows how to get things done. He does not try to impress you with what he's attained, what he has materially—he's just Vinny, a very compassionate, committed man.

When I asked one activist from Maryland what it was like to work with DeMarco, she smiled fondly, took a deep breath, and pronounced, "DeMarco is the world's biggest pain in the ass." When I asked another, she responded simply, "Vinny DeMarco walks with God."

Part I

The Maryland Children's Initiative

In Part I, we learn more about Vincent DeMarco: where he came from, his leadership qualities, his strategic template, his quirks and strengths as leader and strategist. I introduce his closest associates—and most formidable adversaries. I then chronicle a model DeMarco-led campaign, integrating virtually all of his signature organizing skills and strategic innovations.

1

Rescuing a Lost Cause

A Tobacco Lobbyist's Dream

Maryland is a tobacco state—a historic tobacco state, if not a Big Tobacco state. Carved tobacco leaves adorn the balcony railing in Maryland's historic Old Senate Chamber. When the State House was built in the 1770s, tobacco was a form of currency as well as Maryland's major crop. The Great Seal of Calvert County (via Lord Calvert), adopted officially in 1954, features a tobacco leaf, representing the county's leading product. In 2007, the seventy-second Queen Nicotina, selected from local outstanding high school seniors, reigned over the annual Charles County Fair.

But despite the state's tobacco history, from 1992 to 1996, Maryland public health advocates under the umbrella of the Smoke Free Maryland Coalition campaigned to raise the state's thirty-six-cents-per-pack cigarette tax by one dollar. Each year the legislature slammed the door shut on any cigarette tax increase. In 1997, when the coalition tried again, Maryland had barely more than a thousand tobacco farmers. But those farmers and wholesalers from rural southern Maryland had long held the fierce loyalty of the state Senate president, Mike Miller, who vigorously opposed all constraints on tobacco because, he often said, he was raised "surrounded by tobacco fields."

Along with Miller, the tobacco farmers and wholesalers could count on powerful senior legislators from neighboring tobacco-growing districts. From non-tobacco-growing districts, they could count on state legislators who depended on the goodwill of Miller for their rise through the Senate's hierarchy—or who dreaded finding themselves with dead-end committee assignments, no help for a needed bridge or repaved road in their district, and a windowless Senate office in Annapolis, perhaps in the basement of what later was to be immortalized as "the Mike Miller Building."

Outside the legislature, but intimately connected to it, was Bruce Bereano, the veritable dean of Maryland's lobbying corps. A lobbyist for the Tobacco Institute for more than twenty years, Bereano had served as chief of staff to Steny Hoyer (who became Democratic majority leader of the U.S. House of Representatives in 2006) when Hoyer was president of the Maryland Senate. Bereano was close to the governor and virtually every legislative leader in the state. So formidable was he that not even a 1994 criminal conviction could slow him down. To *Washington Post* reporter Daniel LeDuc in February 1997, Senate President Miller clucked appropriate dismay at Bereano's foul play but confessed, "I'd be less than candid if I didn't say he was one of my closest friends."

For wary members of the Maryland legislature, supporting new cigarette taxes in 1997 would mean bucking the 1990s anti-tax tide. In 1992, angry voters had denied the first President George Bush a second term after he broke his pledge ("Read my lips") never to raise taxes. In Maryland, as elsewhere, Democrats and Republicans alike were vowing no tax increases—ever. They were not making fine distinctions, for example, weighing the relative merits of cigarette taxes or the extent of public acceptance of them. Among them was Democrat Mike Miller, who quite aside from his tobacco allegiances was determined to head off Republican broadsides at tax-and-spend Democrats by swearing never to raise any taxes. On a personal level, legislators who were still confirmed smokers viewed cigarette tax increases with their own smoke in their eyes. Their subjective stance offset the personal commitment to tobacco control measures of tobacco's victims and their supporters, among them Democratic governor Parris Glendening, who ached to support a cigarette tax increase as both a health measure and a revenue measure. His mother had died from smoking-inflicted lung cancer.

In 1994—the year Republicans stormed to control of Congress, in no small part by vowing to cut taxes—Glendening had squeaked by in his election by barely five thousand votes over an anti-tax Republican, Ellen Sauerbrey. The new governor had taken comfort in even this narrow victory; he told the *Baltimore Sun*: "We survived a national tide. We're one of the few Democrats who won, one of the few Democratic candidates for governor who won, and one of the very few non-incumbents to win." Now Sauerbrey was on the prowl for issues to spark a rematch in 1998, eyeing Glendening's every action for an opening—a political reality that threatened to sap the governor's enthusiasm for a tobacco tax increase.

If these weren't reasons enough for lobbyist Bereano and Big Tobacco to rest easy, by 1998 Maryland would be looking at a huge budget surplus—close to $1 billion by 1999—boosted by an anticipated windfall from the state attorneys general settlement of their lawsuits against the tobacco companies. Now it would be uphill work for anyone to argue that raising the tax on tobacco would yield both health benefits and needed revenues, the win-win arguments that in 1992 had propelled the last, modest tobacco tax increase. In 1997, once again, tobacco lobbyist Bereano would make certain that no significant cigarette tax increase passed. "I worked with the RJ [R. J. Reynolds Tobacco Company] lobbyist, with the Philip Morris lobbyist," he told me, "and we had that thing dead in the water, dead in the water."

The Health Police: "Sucker-Punched"

In the culmination of their effort in 1997 to get a tobacco tax increase passed, Smoke Free Maryland Coalition strategists packed the House and Senate committee hearings with celebrity witnesses—among them, Maryland's secretary of health, the state attorney general, Pulitzer Prize–winning civil rights historian Taylor Branch, and the Baltimore Orioles team physician. To no avail.

After the coalition went down to defeat on March 31, 1997, C. Fraser Smith, the *Baltimore Sun*'s preeminent political columnist, laid into the health lobbyists and their strategies in a piece headlined "Foes of Tobacco Lost Big—Again; All-or-Nothing Tactics, Some Say, Got Them 'Sucker-Punched.'" Smith narrated a tale of the health advocates' clumsy and uncompromising zealotry: "Partly because health advocates insisted on a whole legislative loaf—they are headed home with none. The health advocates insisted on amending the bill to impose a full dollar-a-pack increase—and lost everything." An official close to the advocates' top political ally, Governor Glendening, lamented their tactics: "They have one play in their playbook: a 100-yard, Hail Mary pass play for a touchdown. They have no other way of getting points on the board."

Smith pointed out that the smoking foes had few personal relationships with committee members, contrasting the insider access of "the pro-tobacco team" with the anti-tobacco lobbyists' outsider status: "Personal relationships are coin of the realm in Annapolis. Veteran lobbyists have been full-service friends to senators or delegates they sometimes refer to as 'votes,' vacationing with them, handling a divorce, playing golf and advising on legislation." The pro-tobacco team, Smith went on, "much larger even than it seems, is disciplined, full-time, tightly meshed and reaching beyond ... the big leagues of cigarette manufacturing. Each one of these lobbyists had his own relationships, too." The columnist cited the political wisdom of Bereano, "one of the longest-serving industry representatives," who told him that "the anti-smoking advocates (he calls them 'health police')" never connected their conceptual case against smoking to the tax increase. Finally, Smith quoted one of the moderate "swing" legislators, Democrat Kumar P. Barve, who mourned, postmortem: "I've never seen so many liberals get sucker-punched on a bill."

While Smith was not unsympathetic to the cause of tobacco control and the boon to health that a tax increase promised, his comparison was unduly harsh to the Smoke Free Maryland Coalition. This was no gang that couldn't shoot straight. Only three years earlier the coalition had won some important state and local battles for smoke-free air. Its core staff members were streetwise and strategic. Its executive director, Kari Appler, housed in the Maryland Medical Society, was a savvy advocate. The coalition organizer, Glenn Schneider, who had recently come from the Maryland Department of Health, was a quick learner and born strategist. Its chief lobbyist, Eric Gally, had lobbied effectively in the legislature for the American Cancer Society in Maryland for years. In Annapolis, though, the coalition was up against a reinforced roadblock, and by 1997 coalition members knew it. Sure, they had made mistakes, but not even a flawless conventional public health campaign could have moved Bereano/Miller & Co. They needed something different.

Why Vincent DeMarco?

Vincent DeMarco had first come to public notice in a *Baltimore Sun* editorial on December 31, 1988, under the headline "Marylander of the Year." The editorial began: "Beyond doubt the most important contribution to the well being and pride of Marylanders in 1988 was the enactment of the Saturday night special law and its endorsement by the voters in a referendum." The so-called Saturday night specials were cheap, short-barreled, lightweight, readily available handguns made of poor-quality materials. Inaccurate and unreliable, they were still deadly. Working with the attorney general and his staff, DeMarco drafted legislation to ban these weapons; the Maryland General Assembly enacted it in 1988, and the referendum upheld the ban.

The *Sun* editorial cited many prominent Marylanders who had contributed to this victory but focused on "the spear-carriers who did the job day to day to get the law and the referendum passed." Foremost among those spear carriers was the *Sun*'s Marylander of the Year, a young junior lawyer in the state attorney general's office, Vincent DeMarco, who "provided backup to all other efforts. He reached out to involve community leaders. He is one of the very few people who believed, from the outset, the fight for a Saturday Night Special Ban could be won."

DeMarco—to this day embarrassed by and uncomfortable with the *Sun's* selection—credits that referendum campaign with teaching him how to put together "an intense coalition" that for the first time tapped the power of an aroused community. Although DeMarco acknowledges that he was "in way over my head, overseeing the media, the polling, the fund-raising," his ally in that campaign, political strategist Bernie Horn, pinpoints DeMarco's unique contribution: "He didn't know anything about polling or media or much else. But he did two very important things." One was that he kept everybody going forward when they "could have formed a circle and shot at each other," Horn said. "And he just made sure that each individual person thought he or she was important, and kept them going forward." With the media, DeMarco had proved an exceptional spokesman "because he is very authentic and is very comfortable speaking, and interesting things come out of his mouth."

Yet it was not DeMarco's Marylander of the Year award or Saturday-night-special lobbying efforts that most intrigued the Smoke Free Maryland advocates in 1997. It was his most recent victory in the gun control campaign that he waged during the very years Smoke Free Maryland was butting its head against Bruce Bereano in the state legislature. Launched in 1994 and victorious in 1996, DeMarco's campaign persuaded legislators to restrict the rampant sales of handguns in the inner city of Baltimore and elsewhere. Targeting traffickers who imported guns from Maryland to Washington, D.C., for use by criminals, DeMarco also led the battle to restrict the number of handguns that could be sold by any one dealer to any one person, the One Handgun per Month Law, which passed in 1996.

What DeMarco could bring to the coalition, its staff thought, in addition to lobbying skills and a network of relationships, was his experience and skill in mobilizing the broad but unfocused popular will. The group knew that the public supported cigarette tax increases and they knew how to lobby, they thought, but they agreed with Eric Gally when he told them: "Vinny is the master of the rest of Maryland. We need him."

By the summer of 1997, DeMarco was more than ready to come to the aid of Smoke Free Maryland. He had become increasingly restless in his role at Handgun Control, Inc., in Washington (later renamed the Brady Campaign). At the national gun control organization inspired by former Ronald Reagan press secretary Jim Brady, for two and a half years he had led the effort to put together a national network of state gun control organizations. The mission had appealed to him—the chance to adapt on a national scale the lessons and strategies he had developed in Maryland. Indeed, he had helped build a formidable coalition of national organizations that defeated an effort by the Republican Congress (elected in 1994 with potent NRA political support) to repeal the assault weapons ban enacted during the Clinton administration.

Over time, though, DeMarco's deeply personal style of operating was not a comfortable fit in a large, bureaucratic organization, where his energy and enthusiasm made others feel uneasy, even threatened. He was not prepared for the sometimes mean-spirited infighting that resulted or for the absence of the collegial support he had enjoyed in his Maryland work. Each day's commute from Baltimore to Washington propelled him from the comfort of his home community into the alien atmosphere of D.C.

So it was with relief and no little excitement that DeMarco received the invitation from Eric Gally to explore a collaboration that would look at reviving Smoke Free Maryland's moribund campaigns to raise the cigarette excise tax. Gally recalls telling DeMarco, "We need somebody in the real world, kicking up the dust."

Can You Believe This Guy?

Gally and the other Smoke Free Maryland staff members briefed DeMarco on their frustrated tax campaign and invited him to meet with and present to the Smoke Free Maryland Board his suggestions for overcoming the legislative obstacles that had thus far bedeviled them. But how would the mostly staid members of the board react to an unconventional dust-kicker? DeMarco met the coalition board and staff at the sober offices of the Maryland Medical Society. To the thirteen or fourteen in the room, DeMarco confidently laid out his proposal for a campaign that incorporated the innovations he had experimented with in his gun control work. Glenn Schneider remembers that meeting "like it was yesterday. People said, 'Yes, we do need to do more; we need to reach out more to the groups that we haven't worked with before; we do have to reach out to the faith community. This is a great idea.'"

Then, Schneider said, DeMarco "dropped a bomb"—his estimate of how much money the coalition would need to get a large tax increase enacted: hundreds of thousands of dollars. The board members were incredulous. Where would such unimagined campaign funds come from? As soon as DeMarco left, Schneider recalls, the board members turned to each other, in wonderment, asking, "Can you believe this guy?" Yet the coalition had no feasible alternative. In the days following the meeting, the staff kept talking about DeMarco and his plan, and the consensus began to shift toward willingness, Schneider said, to "at least give it a shot." The board members agreed—in principle.

But soon, doubts again crept in. "We worried," Schneider recalls, "that we really knew very little about Vinny and how he operated. He had no experience or repute as a tobacco control advocate. What if we're unleashing a loose cannon?" Would DeMarco adhere to the coalition's conviction that its strongest arguments came from the behavioral science that demonstrated the effectiveness of sudden, large leaps in tobacco taxes in reducing teen smoking? In the heat of the legislative session, would he take it upon himself to negotiate compromises without adequate consultation? Would he so dominate media coverage as to eclipse the work of the coalition and its leaders? Concern escalated. The leaders of the voluntary heart, lung, and cancer health associations that were the mainstays of the Smoke Free Coalition conjured up specters of DeMarco poaching for funds on the very individuals and foundations the coalition relied on for its own funding. Mindful of DeMarco's uncanny ability to draw media attention, the last thing it wanted to do was create a competitor.

As fearful as the proverbial woman invited to dance with the eight-hundred-pound gorilla, a three-member committee tackled these concerns by drafting a tough Memorandum of Understanding to present to DeMarco to sign. Schneider elaborates on the concerns that provoked the memorandum:

> We figured that Vinny would only temporarily be a tobacco advocate. We worried that he'd take over the movement by storm, run the campaign independent from us, perhaps negotiate a weaker deal than we'd be comfortable with, claim credit for "success" and leave the movement. Smoke Free Maryland was the only group who'd stick around to finish the job of smoke-free air, et cetera. If we invested resources on this tobacco tax campaign without getting stronger, creating new relationships and getting co-credit for the win, then why do it? We needed Vinny to help us get stronger.

The memorandum would leash DeMarco, Schneider said: "Every time you do a media event, we have to be included. Every time you talk to a reporter, you have to tell him or her to call us. When you go out and meet with people, we want to be involved. If there's a secret meeting, you need to let us know and include us. When you negotiate with major groups, we need to be on board."

When Schneider and his fellow staff members met with DeMarco in a small restaurant and bookstore in downtown Baltimore to present their memorandum, they worried he might balk at the litany of proposed constraints. Schneider still marvels that DeMarco "didn't bat an eye. He said, 'Well, of course. Yes, I can do that. This is easy. I'll sign it.'" They had begun to learn what it meant to work with DeMarco. Over the next months and years, they would learn more, much more.

Where Did He Come From?

Schneider and DeMarco's new colleagues would soon learn where DeMarco came from, both literally and figuratively, and what moved him. The short answer was the town of Trevico, Italy. He was born in 1957 in this small mountain town about one hundred kilometers east of Naples—a town with a view so glorious that the Roman poet Horace hailed the scene from its mountain top as one of the most glorious in all of Italy. The birth was a signal event in the town, recalls DeMarco's mother, Rosa. She relates that the entire town came out to view her first-born and, she maintains, remarkable infant. "When did you know," I asked her, "that Vinny was going to become a special person?" "Before he was born!" she declared without hesitation. Pride? Rosa DeMarco insisted that the right photograph to grace the cover of this book should be the prize photograph of DeMarco standing nobly in front of the White House when the national assault weapons ban was signed into law by President Bill Clinton. She firmly believes that he is a born leader who belongs on the inside of that house. DeMarco muses: "I'll never forget the day I'm six, seven years old, must have been second or third grade . . . when I came home from school and I said to my mother, 'I can't be president, because you have to be born here.' She said, 'We're going to change that law!'"

After the family immigrated to New Jersey in 1961, Rosa, along with her husband, Antonio, worked very hard to make a good life for their children, including providing them with as much education as possible. Rosa worked as a seamstress and was a member of the textile workers union. Antonio worked long overtime hours on the docks as a crane mechanic and belonged to the longshoremen's union. While at work one day, Antonio DeMarco earned the deep respect of his fellow workers by adroitly manipulating the cranes he repaired to save several workers who had fallen into the waters of New York Harbor.

DeMarco learned much from both of his parents about the importance of hard and skillful work and helping others. But he also learned that good work was not automatically rewarded in the United States; it had to be fought for. DeMarco recalls joining his father on the union picket line at age nine when the formidable longshoremen's union was fighting for good pay and health benefits. In college he volunteered to work for the national labor boycott of J. P. Stevens, a textile firm infamous for punishing workers who sought to unionize; and when he later joined a law firm, he urged his fellow employees to join a union, a quixotic effort that the firm successfully stonewalled.

"Quixotic" is a label not infrequently applied by others to DeMarco's ventures, but also one that speaks to his vision of himself. On the landing of the

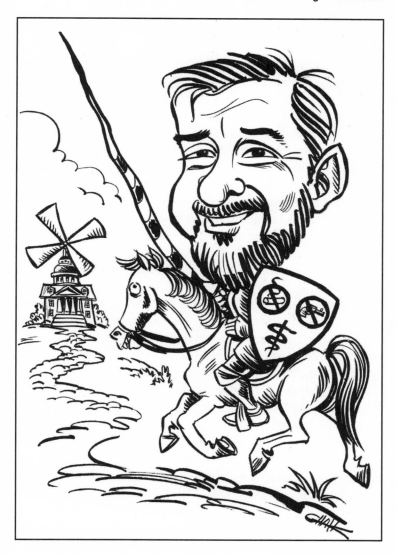

stairway to his offices stands a weather-scarred, three-foot-high lawn sculpture of Don Quixote (that his wife, Molly Mitchell, firmly refused to house inside their home). DeMarco and his younger son Jamie read Cervantes' annals of the Don's misbegotten campaigns together, and the twelve-year-old Jamie would belt out the hero's call to arms against the windmills from the musical version, *The Man of La Mancha*.

When not reading Cervantes, DeMarco reads history. He's drawn to biographies of his heroes, from Franklin and Eleanor Roosevelt to Robert Kennedy and Martin Luther King Jr., who, like Don Quixote, struggle to make impossible dreams realities.

The Catholic Church under Pope John XXIII, with its emphasis on social justice, so influenced the young DeMarco that by the time he reached high school he was determined to enter the priesthood. An intense debate with a Jewish friend, a skeptical fellow ninth grader, he recalls, triggered his increasing doubts about religious dogma. "Though I no longer wanted to be a priest," he says, "the desire to make a difference in society became even stronger." (He and his wife Molly became members of a local Quaker Meeting, where, Molly says, "The focus on 'letting your life speak' and the testimonies of peace, truth, simplicity and equality resonated with us.")

In 1973, as a high school senior in Hazlet, New Jersey, DeMarco launched his first advocacy campaign. As acting mayor for a day in a civics class exercise, he persuaded his student colleagues, sitting as the Township Council, to pass a ban on smoking in the council hearing room where they were meeting. After the vote, DeMarco firmly told the principal, who was still smoking, to put out his cigarette or leave the room. The principal grimly snuffed out his cigarette. The local newspaper's report of the event now hangs in the den in Rosa and Antonio DeMarco's home in Colts Neck, one in a dense display of photographs, clippings, certificates, plaques, awards, and trophies that stretches across two walls, alongside the not inconsiderable memorabilia of DeMarco's accomplished brother Nicola and sisters, Brunella, a social worker, and Marlana, a high school Italian teacher. (These include a news clip on how Nicola, who spent several years in Africa in the Peace Corps working on HIV/AIDS prevention, helped to organize a successful campaign to restore a monument stolen from Ethiopia by Benito Mussolini.)

At Johns Hopkins University, DeMarco took his studies more seriously than most. His Hopkins roommate, Bernie Horn, viewed him with no little awe:

> Vinny and I were together in a class on political theory. It was contemporary political theory, and the professor was Richard Flathman. This was a very difficult course even though the twenty-five of us were mostly political science majors. There's nothing solid about political science, it's about language: What does the word "authority" really mean philosophically?
>
> We would go to class every week. Dr. Flathman would start asking questions, and twenty-four of us could not understand the question. Vinny would answer. Dr. Flathman would ask another question. No one else would understand it. Vinny would answer. It was a two-hour class. So once a week, on Thursdays, I spent listening to Dr. Flathman and Vinny talk to each other.

DeMarco did not spend his time at Hopkins entirely in his head. While there as an undergraduate and then back in graduate school studying American history, he was drawn to the Hopkins Tutorial Project, which had been founded in the 1960s by Hopkins chaplain and Baltimore civil rights leader Rev. Chet Wickwire. His favorite tutee was Eric Anderson, whom he first won over with the magic of Abbott and Costello's "Who's on First" comedy routine. With DeMarco's help, Anderson became a motivated and successful student, graduated from college, and got a job as a benefits technical examiner in the Social Security Administration. DeMarco says he learned much from Anderson, particularly about how to face adversity when he saw Anderson's determination to overcome a nearly fatal brain aneurism when he was a teenager. DeMarco now enjoys sharing the "Who's on First" routine with Anderson's three kids.

But what most engaged DeMarco at Hopkins, and most shaped his future life, was hands-on politics. At Hopkins, DeMarco and a small band of close friends who met through the college debate team became not only roommates but also successive leaders of Maryland's Young Democrats. Instead of dedicating themselves to sports or partying, on their own initiative they conceived, planned, and lobbied for a series of remarkably successful state legislative campaigns, rotating leadership roles.

By the time they graduated, they had lobbied a bill through the Maryland state legislature banning a longstanding practice among electoral candidates: buying the support of political organizations, as well as voters, with funds innocently labeled "walkaround money"—essentially, a bribe for votes. Len Lucchi, the Young Democrats' chief lobbyist, played the lead role in the Hopkins students' effort. Bernie Horn, another core member of this team, remembers: "Len miraculously enacted the law banning walkaround money—one of the biggest bombshells. Len took a bill that was intended to do something else and got it amended. This passed. Len was nobody." Meanwhile, frustrated with weak enforcement of labor protection laws at the federal level, DeMarco as an undergraduate drafted a bill in the late 1970s to prohibit the state government from contracting with companies that violated national labor laws, and then turned to Horn and Lucchi for tactical help. The Maryland General Assembly voted the bill into law in late 1978.

Working on these issues, and drawn from an early age to labor causes, DeMarco developed close ties with labor union lobbyists and experienced firsthand the power of strong coalitions. In 1983 and 1984, along with Lucchi and Horn, he collaborated with the Maryland AFL-CIO to try to persuade the legislature to repeal a resolution it had previously passed that called for a national constitutional convention. The resolution's goal—to require a balanced federal budget—would have crippled the nation. Although Maryland never formally rescinded its call for the convention, the impetus for it petered out. For DeMarco, building a strong coalition of labor, faith, and community groups in this effort was his first introduction to the potential for grassroots coalition building.

DeMarco, Horn, and Lucchi have never stopped collaborating. In each of DeMarco's later campaigns, he reached out to them for counsel and for help with specialized tasks. They are, DeMarco says, "always part of my brain trust." Since opening an independent lobbying operation at age twenty-four, Lucchi has evolved into one of the most skillful and strategically canny lobbyists in the state capital. According to Horn, DeMarco is a "fine lobbyist in his way," but Lucchi is a "truly great lobbyist." Where DeMarco's style is "almost a bull in a china shop," Lucchi's approach is "more delicate. When some real lobbying know-how has been needed, he's been the one." Lucchi commands respect even from lobbying archrival Bruce Bereano: "All of the wonderful human characteristics of a person, Len Lucchi has. He's honest, he's trustworthy, he's not about himself, he's a team player. You just make the whole laundry list. All that's Len Lucchi."

Like Lucchi and DeMarco, Horn continued to pursue a career in liberal democratic advocacy. Working for liberal candidates and causes, he proved as innovative a strategist as DeMarco, as well as a capable organizer. His contribution to the new cigarette tax effort would come from his creative talents in conceiving and designing the potent advertisements that would punctuate the campaign at critical junctures.

DeMarco's Smoke Free Maryland colleagues need not have worried about DeMarco running roughshod over them. From DeMarco's first days as an advocate, his efforts had been collaborative, centering on the complementary skills of the Hopkins trio of campaign-addicted—and skillful—activists. In every campaign in which DeMarco had played a leadership role, he expanded the core team to embrace other advocates with the skills he needed, along with those who best knew the substance of the issue at stake and understood its playing field.

Expanding the Team

As DeMarco assumed the leadership of the cigarette excise tax campaign, he also began to forge close relationships with his new colleagues in tobacco control. He knew he was no public health expert; but Glenn Schneider, by training and experience, was. More than that, public health advocacy was Schneider's calling. He told me: "Much of my passion is faith based (though certainly grounded in science and health policy). Though I don't wear it on my sleeve, my faith is a powerful motivator in my life. My parents taught me by word and example the importance of community service and living out my faith." Schneider has, says DeMarco, "an uncanny ability to make complex matters understandable to most people." Moreover, he would match DeMarco's infectious exuberance with his own booming effervescence. I found no one who was not also disarmed by Schneider's patent integrity. He would prove impossible to dislike, even for those who could not relate to DeMarco's intensity.

DeMarco particularly wanted a team member who could help him reach out to the faith community in Maryland. Bishop Douglas Miles, a friend from gun control days, suggested his wife, Rosanna, and "we hit it off right away," says DeMarco, who hired her as deputy director. It would be another right match, for Rosanna Miles would be instrumental in opening doors for the campaign with faith groups that she and her husband had been working with for years, as well as with Baltimore City elected officials, most of whom the two had known for decades. Schneider and Miles would comprise the core team that came together to develop the tax campaign. Each would be, as DeMarco notes, "involved in all the key decisions."

Living and Working with DeMarco

DeMarco doesn't *look* like a lobbyist, much less like a politician. He's disheveled. He's rumpled. For years in the lobbies of Annapolis, day after day, DeMarco wore for good luck a steadily deteriorating Winnie the Pooh tie that his sons had given him. Former governor Parris Glendening, an ally, would grow so tired of that tie that he seized the occasion of a ceremony celebrating the tobacco tax increase campaign to present DeMarco with an elegant (clean) replacement emblazoned with the seal of Maryland. Then, "to keep the good luck going," DeMarco wore *that* tie day in and day out until Rosanna Miles made him get it cleaned.

He doesn't behave like a lobbyist, either. He doesn't take legislators to lunch, though he takes everyone he can to the Yabba Pot, a Caribbean vegan café down the street from his office, where he recommends the barbecued tofu ribs. His favorite foods are pasta with homemade tomato sauce, hot chocolate with soymilk, vegetable sushi, and miso soup. A labor leader ally once demanded at a roast of DeMarco: "An Italian that is a Quaker that doesn't smoke or drink or eat meat or swear? Who the hell is this guy?!"

Tobacco lobbyist Bruce Bereano operates out of an elegant townhouse near the Capitol and drives his Mercedes to host a lunch at an upscale restaurant for two former governors. DeMarco lives and works simply. His office doesn't look like that of a lobbyist. The space is spare, for a long time furnished in second-hand utilitarian, now simply functional. He once found two office chairs discarded on the street down the block and brought them in. When one group of interns left, inspired by their experience but aching from the ancient, malformed office chairs, they presented to DeMarco, as their parting gift, a brand-new ergonomic office chair.

Most community organizers are single-minded in pursuit of their social justice passions. For DeMarco, family comes first—Molly and their sons Tony and Jamie. He always does his best to be at all work-related meetings and hearings, but he also is determined to get to as many of his sons' sports games and plays as he can. In an important hearing before the Senate Finance Committee on the 2007 Medicaid expansion law, DeMarco found himself torn between advocacy and family. The hearing had droned on, and DeMarco's scheduled testimony was pushed back until the late afternoon, when his son Tony was about to play in a championship high school basketball game. DeMarco would not wait. He asked his colleague Len Lucchi to testify for him while he quietly ducked out to the game.

His ability to engage even reluctant allies in active participation in his campaigns reflects not only his relentlessness, but his skill. Kathleen Kennedy Townsend, the former lieutenant governor of Maryland, who had known and supported DeMarco from his first years of campaigning, recalls his early days:

> When I first met Vinny, he was like many young people I was meeting in 1982: focused on bringing nuclear weapons to a halt, and very passionate about what he was doing. He had organized a group of Young Democrats to come to the nuclear freeze march in New York. And I saw that passion. Since then, he's focused very deeply on one critical issue after another, whether it be guns or tobacco or health care.

She speaks movingly of her response to DeMarco's call for help at the height of his campaign against Saturday-night-special handguns. DeMarco had succeeded in lobbying the ban on such guns through the legislature, but the NRA had launched a voter referendum campaign to overturn the legislation. Townsend notes that the 1968 gunshot assassination of her father Robert Kennedy was still raw when DeMarco asked her to sign a letter in 1988 in opposition to the referendum:

> I had never spoken about guns before that. It was too painful for me to speak about it; too awful and sad. But when Vinny asked me, I said yes. I had never said yes to anybody before. But he also made it easy. I remember he brought me the letters; he gave them to me, I just signed them. He would describe

to the world, "How incredible it is that Kathleen did all this work!" In fact, I didn't really do anything. He did it all.

He gives you credit. He makes you feel good. You feel that he's going to protect you in any way he can. In the end, we all love Vinny. But at the moment, he's being very solicitous about my time, my feelings, what's going on in my life. So he realizes—which is the great thing about a leader—that he's in there for the long haul, not for the day.

Molly Mitchell

Molly Mitchell and DeMarco met while campaigning for liberal Steve Sachs in his unsuccessful run for governor of Maryland in 1986. They were working the streets of Baltimore in a neighborhood of students and young professionals. "I remember watching Vinny," Mitchell says. "We were handing out literature to people on the streets. I'd look at people and see if they were making eye contact with me. Only if they seemed interested would I hand them something. But Vinny would just walk up to anybody, no matter what, thrust the handout in their hands and say, 'Here—here's Steve Sachs!'" In a mingling of Italian slang and Yiddish, she recalls with a grin: "I just thought, this guy is really what his parents would call a *facia tosta* [roughly translated, an "in-your-face guy"]. He's got a lot of—I don't know—chutzpah."

Like DeMarco, Mitchell was drawn to social justice activism while still in college. She was studying geography at the University of West Virginia when she took a summer job in her hometown, Baltimore, canvassing door-to-door for the Maryland Citizen Labor Energy Coalition. She then sought an internship to stay on and helped mobilize more than five hundred people to protest at a hearing against a utility rate increase.

After college she stayed in West Virginia for two years, first as a community organizer for the West Virginia Citizen Action Group on energy and environmental issues, then running the door-to-door state senate campaign for the group's founder, David Grubb. With some fellow organizers, she went down to North Carolina to support the Democratic primary campaign of a candidate who would have been the first African American to represent that state since Reconstruction.

Back in Maryland, Mitchell and DeMarco found a spiritual home in a Quaker Meeting and were married in a Quaker ceremony. (I was impressed when, years later, a Methodist leader spoke of how moved she was by DeMarco's insistence on beginning meetings with other faith leaders with a Quaker prayer. Upon reflection, I challenged DeMarco when next we met: "There are no Quaker prayers!" He responded without hesitation, "I simply ask for a moment of silence.") Mitchell earned a law degree and went on to work on public health policy issues, such as alcohol problems, for then lieutenant governor Kathleen Kennedy Townsend.

"I think I've always had a really strong sense of justice," Mitchell reflects. "I always wanted to do something that was going to make a difference. Part of it was growing up Catholic, just taking very seriously that 'whatever you do to each of my brothers, that you do unto me.'" This is no small commitment on her part; she has five brothers and five sisters.

Mitchell is characteristically modest about her role in DeMarco's campaigns; she doesn't see herself as a member of his "brain trust": "I see myself playing a role of personal support, sounding board, and witness to all of this." DeMarco insists that "Molly is greatly understating the key role she has always played as part of the brain trust on all these adventures. We always discuss everything we're doing." Len Lucchi confirms this: "He bounces ideas off her all the time."

Mitchell is even-keeled and warm, but sober in contrast to DeMarco's restless energy. DeMarco can be impulsive; Mitchell is always reflective. Both are often funny, but Mitchell's wit is contained, while DeMarco is prone to bouts of infectious laughter. Of Mitchell, Townsend says: "Molly is the classic ideal of a wise woman. She was my aide-de-camp when I first ran for lieutenant governor. I had two people whom I would drive around with. Because I was so busy, I couldn't do with just one, it would have been too much. But David, my husband, always said 'Ah' when I came home with Molly. I was so much happier."

DeMarco says of his wife: "She's a bulwark for me in times of stress and an inspiration in times of hope."

Flaws and Foibles

Through the years and campaigns since they teamed up at Johns Hopkins, Lucchi and Horn have learned to prize DeMarco's strengths and to tolerate his undeniably maddening idiosyncrasies. Lucchi laments: "His hair is always askew. When he comes to Annapolis to lobby, the first thing I do is hand him a comb." On the rare occasions when DeMarco must dress for an important occasion such as a hearing or a press conference, he wears for good luck the suit he was married in back in 1987. He often appears hopelessly disorganized. "He uses a tourist bag instead of a briefcase," Lucchi says, "so every paper he hands to someone is always dog-eared. His staff tries to keep handouts away from him and in file folders."

Staffer Matt Celentano vents his frustration with DeMarco's disorganization: "He's always losing stuff. He constantly steals office supplies, so we have to hide them from him—it's unbelievable. His glasses, though, are the worst thing. He has five or six pair in the office, and he *still* can't find them. And when he does, they're generally broken, and he sometimes wears them broken!" "His enthusiasm is unnatural," claims Bernie Horn. "His energy is unnatural." A night owl, Horn recalls with a shudder the many mornings DeMarco, his Hopkins roommate, blasted him from sleep at daybreak singing operatic arias. DeMarco is enthusiastic even in his frustration, says staffer Rosanna Miles. "Vinny will get over to the copier machine and just tear it up. He'll yell, 'What's wrong with this machine! Where's Glenn?' He's not a person that likes to deal with what he sees as insignificant things. If the phone, if his computer, isn't working, oh God, he goes crazy. He's not a fixer, not with his hands."

DeMarco drives even his fondest colleagues crazy with his communications madness. As Celentano says:

> He has to be in constant communication, and if he's not, he gets all flustered. When I first got here, he was all pager. He would get paged and he would scream and run away, and you wouldn't know what he was going for. Then he went to BlackBerry, which he proceeded to destroy, because he did about sixteen hundred one-word e-mails a day on it. . . . Then he went to this cell phone. Now he will routinely be answering the cell phone while on the work phone at the same time and have a call waiting, and he tries to do all three at once.

Eric Gally describes a scenario he imagines occurring when DeMarco's name shows up on someone's caller ID: "People will yell, 'Look, it's Vinny again! Who wants to talk to Vinny?' I'm sure some people give their phone to their kids and let him talk to them." Of the machine-gun fire of e-mails and smartphone missiles that issue from DeMarco, Lucchi adopts the only defense available: "The only way I can make sure that my BlackBerry does not fill up on e-mails is to have him at my side so he can't send any; ditto for voice mails."

Rosanna Miles's first encounter with DeMarco was not when he interviewed her for the job, but several years earlier when he was desperate to produce busloads of volunteers to swarm the legislature in Annapolis in support of yet another gun control measure. Her husband Bishop Miles had suggested that his wife could help, and she and DeMarco met for lunch. Miles recalls that DeMarco buried his head in his food and, without looking up, bluntly demanded, "How many buses can you deliver?" Though she ultimately delivered three forty-two-passenger busloads, she complained to her husband that his friend was "a very strange guy." DeMarco's recollection that he and Rosanna Miles "hit it off right away" is not exactly Miles's recollection. As she once said, "He has a convenient forgettery."

Further confusion arose when Miles first reported to her new job. DeMarco had not told her exactly what her duties were (and he never would). So she asked the only employee hired before her, Rev. Linda Coveleskie, who responded, "I have no idea, either." His colleagues would encounter other vexing frustrations: DeMarco could unexpectedly prove relentlessly stubborn. Once he had determined a course of action, his usually sunny mood could swing from what one staff member calls his "reckless optimism" to gloomy pessimism. On the reckless optimism front, DeMarco's vision of the attainable could flummox his colleagues, such as his publicly announcing a large media event with no consultation and no conceivable time for the staff to organize it—though, more often than not, they succeeded, breathlessly.

DeMarco's fierce loyalty to longtime friends and allies could blur his judgment, as Rosanna Miles illustrates: "Glenn and I would say to him, about a friend who has persuaded DeMarco to follow a wrong-headed strategy or tactic, 'This person is not showing that he is on our side, and you can't continue to go in that direction, no matter what the person has done for you before.' He will go the distance with persons that he cares about and not question their ability—it is enough that the person is a friend."

Yet Nobody Ever Quits

"Vinny's such a whirlwind," Molly Mitchell says of her husband, "and he thinks he can just give people a word or two, 'Do this!' and 'Do that!' and they're going to know what they have to do. Some of the people that worked under him felt like he just didn't give them enough direction, that they were left on their own and didn't know what they were supposed to be doing." Mitchell laughs. "You've heard people say he drives them crazy? He drives *everybody* crazy. He's so disorganized." But the "amazing thing," she quickly adds, "is that it doesn't interfere with his getting things done. *He* knows what he's doing." Glenn Schneider agrees: "Vinny is always clear about our mission. There is never a day that we don't understand the gist of what he wants. We just have trouble operationalizing those desires." To fill this gap, DeMarco recruits colleagues who not only complement his skills, but also compensate for his flaws, as Bernie Horn observes: "Vinny'd probably make a great CEO of a big company, because he's great at delegating. He's great at understanding who's good at what and what to trust people with."

DeMarco's choice of campaign deputy, Glenn Schneider, demonstrates this quality. Schneider is as organized in office matters as DeMarco is disorganized; as at home with the new technologies as DeMarco is initially thwarted by them; as patient as DeMarco is impatient. The many papers and computer files DeMarco loses, Schneider finds. As mindful of the human needs of fellow workers as DeMarco was preoccupied with the needs of the campaign, Schneider became DeMarco's indispensable right arm. As Schneider reads him, DeMarco often has a hard time figuring out "what people power is needed to accomplish certain tasks or whether a timeline he sets is realistic, or the priority steps we needed to take before moving on to another priority, or what our staff or volunteers need to effectively complete the task." As Schneider points out, "That's why you have a solid team that can translate Vinnyspeak into smooth operations."

After meetings in which DeMarco told the staff what he wanted done, Schneider says, staffers and interns would sit down and discuss how to deal with a laundry list of often competing priorities. "I remember meetings with Rosanna and other staff with me starting off saying, 'Okay, let me translate and prioritize the forty things he just asked for.'" For example, Schneider says, DeMarco might say to whatever intern happened to be at hand, without thought to what he or she was already assigned to do, "I need you to call these groups and get them to say yes" to whatever had just come up. Or an intern who had just taken an urgent phone call from Vinny might turn to staff members and ask: "How do I do this? What should I say? Oh, and by the way, I'm here today but I'm not back until next Tuesday. Who should I hand this off to?"

Rosanna Miles has her own method for coping with DeMarco's tendency to issue scattershot directions: "He has so many things in his head that he's trying to put them in place. I've learned how to put his requests in compartments. I can't grasp everything he's running back and forth saying to me, so I have to sift it out in my own mind, though it runs me crazy sometimes." Miles has become the wise heart at the center of the team, "the glue in our organization," says Glenn Schneider. A key reason she is so effective, he believes, is that "she talks about the why of our work and the outcomes of our work in a way that hits home with most." That is, she focuses on and keeps others on the staff "centered on the people we are helping and not the political game that surrounds our work." Miles is "an intuitive, passionate people reader" who not only knows when and how to boost someone's ego but has the grace to do so in the presence of others, Schneider says, "so you feel valued." She discovers a personal connection with almost everyone she meets, and on the rare occasions she feels unsure about someone, her reaction is "one more tool" for Schneider to consider. Finally, "she can put Vinny in his place, and me too. She's the only one who can."

Whatever his management shortcomings, DeMarco's ability to envision realistic paths to change kept his colleagues fully engaged, year after year, as he devised both long- and short-term advocacy strategies. Rosanna Miles and her colleagues may not have known the precise duties of their offices, but they understood enough to go on to build some of the most powerful citizen-based coalitions in Maryland's history.

They were also drawn to DeMarco's unfailing generosity of spirit. Schneider had been used to the order and formality of his previous employers, the state health department and the Medical Society. As he was preparing to join the Health Care for All! campaign, he asked DeMarco what vacation time came with the job. "Whenever you feel you need a vacation," was the answer. "What about sick leave?" asked Schneider. "Whenever you're sick, or there's sickness in the family, stay home." (Of course, he might add, "but when you get back make sure you get those resolutions signed.")

By the fall of 1997, old DeMarco hands and new had come together as the team that would lead the campaign. They were ready to support DeMarco's strengths and accommodate his foibles. They valued his enthusiasm, his strategic sense, his organizing zeal, his network of hundreds of contacts, his media skills. If they did not love his disarray, they prized the opportunity to work with him. Yet even with this impressive core team, how could DeMarco overcome the vast resources and unique access to lawmakers that Bereano and his Big Tobacco allies enjoyed? What political counterweight could DeMarco fashion that would succeed where the fifty-six member groups of the Smoke Free Maryland Coalition had failed?

2

The DeMarco Campaign Template

Policy advocacy campaigns usually follow a customary path: set a legislative objective; call upon known allies to activate an existing coalition, whose leadership signs petitions to the governor and legislators in session; organize from among coalition members supportive letters and e-mails; recruit impressive witnesses to testify before legislative committees; mobilize a few volunteers and one or two paid lobbyists to lobby the legislature; generate some press coverage—perhaps an editorial or two; and, limited funds permitting, buy a few paid ads, all during the legislative session.

The campaign plan DeMarco presented when he first met with the Smoke Free Maryland Board—essentially the plan he was ready to implement—did not just carry a shocking price tag for a public interest campaign. It was a radical departure from any legislative campaign Smoke Free Maryland had engaged in before. It would be more elaborately planned, its time frame longer, each element far more ambitious, and its thrust more aggressively *political.*

This campaign, beginning in mid-1997 and ending with the legislative session, the Maryland General Assembly, in April 1999, would unfold through several overlapping stages. The number and precise nature of these stages would vary from campaign to campaign, but planned staging would be a central element of DeMarco's strategic template in each campaign. Each stage has discrete objectives and strategies:

Stage 1.   Initial organizing of the campaign coalition (summer 1997)
Stage 2.   Opening the conversations with a resolution
Stage 3.   Legislative session trial run (January–April 1998)
Stage 4.   Primary elections and general election candidates pledge campaign (summer and fall 1998)
Stage 5.   Pressure on the legislature for action (January–April 1999)
Stage 6.   Accountability for opponents of tax increase (May 1999)

Integral to each stage, and tailored to each stage, as we shall explore in Chapter 3, would be public education, or, more precisely, media advocacy.

Len Lucchi boils the six stages down to DeMarco's essential strategy, warning that this is "obviously a gross simplification": "He takes a problem, defines the problem, gets those who have power to commit to collusion. He runs a campaign to educate the voting public about it. Then, hopefully, he elects some people in the process. Then, just as important, he holds the people who pledge in the campaign to do the right thing, to stay on board."

During the cigarette tax campaign, DeMarco would use some traditional tactics but, more central to his success, would introduce critical innovations that were not what almost any other experienced advocacy professional would have done.

Given their always scarce funds, most public interest campaigners would have begun by reviewing the readily available public polls demonstrating that cigarette taxes were popular. Despite this ready-made ammunition, DeMarco would engage high-end national pollsters to conduct not just one but three expensive polls in the course of the campaign—and deploy their results in unique ways.

DeMarco wouldn't seek lead partners primarily from among health groups and their customary allies as other tobacco control coalitions had; instead, he would reach out to key allied groups that had never been in the forefront of a tobacco control campaign.

He wouldn't base the excise tax campaign within the Smoke Free Maryland Coalition and its members, the permanent coalition led by the voluntary cancer, lung, and heart associations and the Medical Society—the conventional center of every other state tobacco control campaign; instead, he would create a temporary advocacy organization dedicated solely to this single excise tax campaign, and recruit not individual members but hundreds of community groups and civic associations whose primary interests lay outside health policy advocacy. In this process, he would not shun public alliance with faith leaders and groups, as tobacco control advocates often had (their fear was that such alliances would cause opponents to view them as religious "temperance" zealots, not science-based public health advocates). DeMarco would recruit churches, synagogues, and other faith organizations as his primary political vanguard.

He wouldn't call the new organization something obvious, like the Maryland Cigarette Excise Tax Coalition; instead, he would name it the Maryland Children's Initiative (MCI). He wouldn't beg funding from skittish foundations and other philanthropic sources in return for a pledge to shun political advocacy—the dreaded third rail of tax-exempt foundations; instead, he would convince these foundations that they could fund aggressive public education—which was not, in the legal sense, lobbying—and that they could safely trust him not to cross the legal boundary with their money. (When he did need to cross the line to political activity that philanthropy could not fund, he would raise and safely insulate "hard" political money from "soft" money.)

He wouldn't, in the beginning, seek signatures from potential allies to a letter or petition to lawmakers, or lobby them to support the tax increase in the next session of the legislature; instead, he would at first appear to ignore the legislators altogether. He would simply seek hundreds of potential allies to sign a broad resolution of support for a $1.50-a-pack excise tax increase.

He wouldn't hope to enact a $1.50 tax increase in 1998, in the campaign's first legislative session; instead, he would treat advocacy for the tax increase in that session as a trial run, knowing the effort almost certainly would fail.

He wouldn't wait until the 1999 legislative session to pressure the governor and legislators to support the cigarette tax increase; instead, he would launch an intensely political—though strictly nonpartisan—tax increase campaign focused squarely on the September 1998 state primary elections and the November 1998 state general elections.

He wouldn't turn to a communications specialist to get press coverage for the tax effort after the campaign was designed; instead, he would rely on his own media advocacy skills to gain media coverage, designed from the beginning into each stage of the campaign. He wouldn't hog the headlines, as campaign leaders are tempted to do; instead, he would arrange for every media event to lead with compelling spokespeople ranging from scientifically authoritative medical experts to morally authoritative faith leaders. His name, with a short sound bite framing the campaign's core message for that stage, would be buried somewhere in the middle of virtually every story.

Not one of DeMarco's tactics for gaining the excise tax increase was arbitrary. Most relied on strategies he had tried and tested in his earlier campaigns. Most were embedded in the proposal he presented at his first meeting with the Smoke Free Maryland Board. All responded to the political realities that confronted them.

Stage 1. Initial Organization

Although DeMarco had assured an incredulous Smoke Free Maryland Board that he could raise all the money necessary to conduct a winning campaign, by mid-1997, with the campaign set to launch, he still had no money to support even himself, much less his grandiose plan. He knew, at least, where he could start. The key would be his existing funder base. He would talk first with Robert Embry, president of the Baltimore-based Abell Foundation, a leader admired and followed as both sound and safe by other Maryland philanthropists. It had been Embry who had first sought out DeMarco in 1988, offering to fund his gun control advocacy full time, allowing him to leave his daytime job in the attorney general's office. Over the years, their connection had ripened into deep mutual respect and friendship that DeMarco tended assiduously. The two men spoke often on the phone, exchanging news and insights about the political environment for the social justice issues they both cared about. But mostly what Embry respected about DeMarco was that he consistently delivered on his promises to make policy change happen.

Nonetheless, DeMarco knew Embry would need to be convinced that the tobacco tax campaign was both sound public policy and realistic. Before approaching the philanthropist, he consulted with Carol Beck, a program officer at the Abell Foundation and yet another DeMarco "good friend," who had supported his gun control campaigns. She was very helpful, he notes, "in putting together the proposal in a way that would be appealing to Bob and to the Abell board." But DeMarco took no chances: "I also reached back to my friend Delegate Sandy Rosenberg, in whose office I had my first talk with Bob about gun control fund-raising. Sandy agreed to help me convince Bob that this project made sense." When he finally met with Embry, DeMarco took along Glenn Schneider, counting on his deep knowledge of the health and policy science of tobacco. Schneider confesses to being not a little intimidated by the meeting with so lofty an eminence—literally:

> Here I am, sitting with the CEO of a big foundation in a very impressive twenty-third-floor office overlooking the inner harbor of Baltimore. Embry wants to know everything that's going on and what we're planning. So I'm sitting here with Vinny talking about the policy and politics of the campaign.
>
> After the meeting, Bob Embry e-mails Vinny with hard questions. "Tell me about this," he would write, sending an article from the *Wall Street Journal* lambasting tobacco tax policy. "What do you think?"
>
> Vinny called me up, saying, "You need to convince him that this is an extremely important campaign that we need to do." I felt that same pressure, so I took all the fact sheets and background research we had and put them together bound up in a nice package.

Their combined efforts convinced Embry, and Abell provided the first big grant to the campaign, $90,000. That grant not only would be the cornerstone of the campaign's funding, but also would reassure other potential funders, who might otherwise be intimidated at the prospect of the Internal Revenue Service (IRS) looking over their shoulders and being on the alert for grants that transgressed the gray line between public education and lobbying. Schneider felt reassured, telling himself, "This guy can actually raise some funds." Over the several years of the MCI campaign, DeMarco would raise more than $200,000 in grants from Abell and other foundations with which he had "a good relationship." He would also receive financial support in cash and in kind (for example, paid newspaper ads) from The Robert Wood Johnson Foundation and the national Campaign for Tobacco-Free Kids, as well as from the lead partners in the MCI campaign.

First, We Get Organized

"A great mistake that I see progressive groups making a lot," cautions DeMarco, "is trying to build your coalition during the [legislative] session or right before the session. I believe you need a year or more of getting people invested. So when you want something to happen, these groups are already there. Build that influence up and *then* go to the policymakers—it's much more fruitful."

Put simply, DeMarco and Glenn Schneider set out in their excise tax campaign to build organization power able to jolt the legislature into action when the time was ripe. DeMarco's first order of business was to commission a poll to test the *intensity* of public support for a tax increase. Only fierce, fervent public feeling would motivate voters—and convince elected officials that they would defy such support at their own political peril. In the summer of 1997, DeMarco hired the national Democratic political pollster Celinda Lake, whose polls were respected by and credible among elected officials. As DeMarco hoped—and expected—Lake found overwhelming voter support even for a walloping $1.50-a-pack cigarette tax hike.

While the public's preference was no surprise, DeMarco was buoyed by another of the poll's findings—the "substantial movement in swing voters based on candidates' support for this issue," he said. "This finding laid the groundwork for my belief that this issue, like the gun issue, could play a critical role in the election. And the campaign only works if it can make a difference in an election."

The pre-campaign poll would reap other rewards. Its impressive results would offer powerful persuasion to potential new allies that this was a campaign that could win—despite the prevailing political wisdom. Sharing the poll with potential lead partners "in secret" before it was publicly released helped DeMarco give them a sense of being privileged insiders. When recruitment of these partners reached critical mass and the campaign was ready for a public launch, notes Schneider, "we could announce the statewide results of the poll and subsequently launch the campaign with local results in every part of the state." The public release would yield yet another bonus: even more groups would learn of the poll results and scramble to leap aboard a campaign locomotive now seen to be gathering momentum.

What they would join, however, would not be the Smoke Free Maryland Coalition or the Campaign for a Cigarette Tax Increase, but a new entity that did not even have the words "smoke free" or "tax" in its name. DeMarco was determined from the beginning that he would not serve as a staff member or even the head of Smoke Free Maryland. Instead, he would create a temporary nonprofit organization. Its mission would be singular, its life expectancy short: "Pass the cigarette tax by 1999; then go out of business." This sunset promise went into the new organization's bylaws. As DeMarco and his team set about recruiting partners and allies, the promise would minimize concerns that the new organization would take on permanent life and end up competing with those allies for money. Sun-setting would also allay any fears that DeMarco would soak up media attention forever. Smoke Free Maryland's staff and board members embraced DeMarco's vision. It would keep its separate structure and identity, and the new organization would take the lead, while Cancer Society lobbyist Eric Gally would play a critical supporting role in the lobbying. A new organization would create something the coalition alone could not, said Gally, who saw the two efforts as "the perfect marriage of what we did well in the halls of Annapolis with the traditional health groups that people expected to be lobbying, like the Cancer Society," and of what DeMarco did well, "creating the understanding among legislators that real people out in the real world care about this."

The new organization would need a name. DeMarco and his colleagues pored over the poll data. What leapt out were the most important reasons people supported the tax increase: their beliefs that it would discourage teenagers from smoking and that its proceeds could help fund the urgent needs of children. As Schneider says, the team recognized that "this was all about kids." Horn came up with the name Maryland Children's Initiative. DeMarco seized upon it.

Securing the Base and Recruiting the Lead Organizations

Not that DeMarco would ride off unrestrained under the MCI banner. From the start, he made sure he had a close working relationship with the Smoke Free Maryland staff and board. DeMarco's strategy was to bring the core staff team on board first and then, together with them, meet with the Smoke Free Maryland Board members to present and clear his plans at each stage of the campaign. As he developed tactical initiatives, he would clear these with the board as well. Perhaps most important, his consultations were not window dressing. "He was always open to changing a plan if we objected to a tactic, a strategy, or even terminology," Schneider says. "And because Vinny and I were working so closely together, there was never a time I can remember where he didn't ask for input on even mundane decisions."

In keeping with the Memorandum of Understanding, Smoke Free Maryland would hold a designated seat on the MCI Board. Yet the coalition leaders still did not trust DeMarco completely, Schneider points out, or "why would we need the Memo of Understanding?" The coalition board had veto power over every decision, and they counted on that leverage, he says: "If Smoke Free Maryland ended up distancing itself from the campaign, Vinny would have had a very hard, if not impossible, job ahead of him."

Next, DeMarco would recruit a handful of lead organizations beyond Smoke Free Maryland that would bring critical strengths to the campaign. They could provide new professional lobbying staff, along with engagement in the campaign of grassroots membership. They could bring identification with the issues that the polls showed were most salient for voters. They could bring money, including hard—political—money, and human resources; communications and mobilization networks; and vital media access. They could bring political clout. Their names spread across the MCI logo and banner would signify to all the nature and breadth of support.

How would DeMarco choose which groups to recruit as lead organizations? He and his team turned to the same poll results that had guided their naming of MCI and that pointed to the two benefits of a tax increase that moved voters: higher cigarette taxes were a strong tool for reducing teenage smoking, and the tax revenues generated could strengthen education and meet children's needs in other areas. Thus, the campaign sought as lead partners highly visible, respected groups that the public saw as serving children's needs—including, of course, groups that were also in a position and likely to contribute, as Schneider bluntly acknowledged, "time, talent, and treasure."

The poll results, as hoped, proved a powerful recruiting tool, with their promise of potential victory. But as DeMarco's colleague Bernie Horn points out, it wouldn't be easy:

All these groups have five million demands on them all the time, yet they're always looking for something substantial to engage their members. You need to go to them and talk about the solution, bring them evidence that it works—evidence of how this is working in other states is critical. You need to convince them they can play a big role, that their group can make a difference. Tell them, "We have a plan that can result in a law." Then they're invested in it. They like to be part of something that can win, something they will always be able to tout as an accomplishment, and something that will be good for them institutionally.

Each group MCI approached to be a lead partner was willing to sit down and talk. Each was willing to send senior staff to a large meeting in which DeMarco and his team confidentially shared the poll results. The MCI team gauged each group's interest and its commitment to a leadership role in the campaign. All of them said, according to Schneider, "This is something we really want to get involved with." That was the first step. "We didn't talk yet about how the pie—the funds raised by the tax—would be divided," says Schneider. Once the groups had leapt on board, then they would decide how to split the money.

The health-focused Smoke Free Maryland groups had little experience working with these organizations, and few relationships to build upon. DeMarco had both, which fast-tracked recruiting. For example, he had grown close to the teachers' union president and lobbyists while working with them in his gun control campaigns. Schneider found it "fantastic" that DeMarco had "that kind of access to people who were very powerful outside the scope of our normal health groups."

Critical to the strength of these partnerships was DeMarco's canny grasp of the particular interests of each group. For instance, evidence that raising the cigarette tax was the most effective way to dissuade teenagers from taking up smoking or leading them to quit early carried a great deal of weight with teachers. But at least equally attractive was the campaign poll's revelation that voters liked the idea of applying the tax to children's education needs—smaller classrooms, after-school programs, and, perhaps, higher wages or pensions for teachers. The message was clear, says Schneider: "If you elect lawmakers who care about tobacco taxes, you elect lawmakers who care about teachers."

So it went with each of the other potential lead partners. DeMarco's past networking would open the door. Then Schneider's authoritative science and policy grounding would make the substantive case for the tax increase. Next, DeMarco would highlight the potential benefits for the causes at the top of the organization's priority list and infect the group with his optimism. Each target partner signed on, and each brought needed resources to the common cause—here, money for polling; there, in-kind help such as printing services; and everywhere, enthusiastic, available bodies to amplify the advocacy. Soon he had recruited the five lead partners that MCI needed and that would share equal prominence with Smoke Free Maryland: the Maryland State Teachers Association, Advocates for Children and Youth, the Safe and Sound Campaign (a Baltimore group dedicated to improving conditions for children and youth in the city), the Maryland Association of Student Councils, and Addiction Treatment Advocates of Maryland.

Stage 2. Opening the Conversations with a Resolution

Beyond the lead partners, it was DeMarco's goal to draw into this campaign a far broader, politically influential network of less central allies joined in support of the tobacco tax increase. He would build outward from the base of the fifty or so public health and medical groups that made up the Smoke Free Maryland Coalition and the other lead organizations.

He would not seek, however, to build for MCI itself a large grassroots base of individual members to advocate for the tax increase through calls, letters, demonstrations, and lobbying. Yes, there would be a modest effort to recruit engaged individual activists, but by far his most intense organizing effort would be outreach to the leadership of local and state—and sometimes national—organizations. Once these leaders had enlisted, he would rely on *them* to mobilize their networks of individual members or supporters when action was needed. DeMarco finds this both a more efficient and a more effective strategy, and one that avoids the debilitating effect of real or perceived competition for individual members.

His vehicle for opening this "conversation with the people of Maryland," as he would call it, was a one-page resolution that he asked the leaders of hundreds of community organizations in Maryland to sign on behalf of their group. Not—yet—a commitment to join an organized campaign; not yet a request for a donation; not yet a commitment of time and campaign duties. Just a signature.

Bernie Horn analyzes the thinking behind the resolution, a deceptively simple organizing tool:

> Vinny's real innovation was organizing around a resolution, not a bill. The way policy ordinarily works is that people write a bill, and then they go around to groups saying, "Will you sign on your organization to this bill?" Literally, there's a sign-on letter. Whether they sign on or not depends on the details of the bill. Groups that don't get involved in legislation can't get involved. And the truth is, legislators really don't care much what groups sign on. It doesn't have a substantial impact compared to the kind of thing that Vinny does.
>
> Vinny goes around with a resolution. Any group can agree to a resolution, even those that don't get involved with legislation. They're not committing to lobbying; they're just passing a resolution. The process of passing a resolution activates people. And it gives you access to people. It's a way of introducing yourself, and it's a way of getting people to be a part of your group, and it gives you an excuse to report back to them all the time.

The first task was to develop the precise wording of the resolution, especially the size of the tax increase they would seek and the allocation of the revenues. This process provided the perfect opportunity to demonstrate to the new lead partners, as DeMarco puts it, "true friendship and partnership." With encouragement, all the potential lead organizations agreed—"with varying degrees of enthusiasm"—that they needed to commit to the overriding goal of increasing the tobacco tax to reduce teen smoking. They then worked out together the kind of children-oriented programs that the increase should fund that would drive home the point that this was the Maryland *Children's* Initiative. After some discussion, DeMarco says, they agreed on the core items to be funded, "with each of the lead partners being heavily invested in at least one of these."

The resolution called upon the legislature to:

Increase the Maryland excise tax on cigarettes by $1.50 per pack and extend the tax to other tobacco products

Provide money to fund statewide initiatives that support the healthy development of Maryland's children

Fund a campaign to discourage children from using alcohol, tobacco, and other drugs and to provide treatment for citizens already addicted

Fund a campaign to improve reading among Maryland's public school students, particularly in the elementary grades, by methods such as significantly reducing class sizes

Provide high-quality and affordable child-care and after-school programs for children throughout Maryland

Develop communitywide plans that focus on measurable results and increased opportunity for children

Each organization that signed the resolution would also promise to take two actions. First, it would inform its members and, where possible, the public of its endorsement of the resolution. Second, it would inform the governor, members of the General Assembly, and 1998 candidates for state and local offices of its endorsement of the resolution, to the extent permitted by law, and urge its members to do so also.

A Recruiting Pilgrimage
Now, DeMarco, Schneider, and Miles, with help from the Smoke Free Maryland Coalition staff and leadership, set out on a recruiting pilgrimage to achieve their organizing goal of gathering at least one hundred new signatories to the resolution during the first month. As Schneider says, they "hustled, talking to everyone under the sun to sign on." The result of all this activity and

all the signings was "a mind-boggling number" of groups, says Bernie Horn—ultimately, 365. "Vinny didn't stop at the groups that lobby in Annapolis. He went to the local Cub Scouts, individual churches and synagogues, and local community groups across the state—wherever there were bodies and people who could potentially get activated, he went there."

Highest on DeMarco's campaign plan list was to engage the faith community in tobacco control more deeply than it had ever been before. As a first step, he was determined to recruit Bishop Douglas Miles, pastor of Baltimore's Koinonia Baptist Church and, of course, Rosanna Miles's husband. But, the bishop recalls, "Tobacco was the last thing on my mind, given all the problems Baltimore was facing." Despite Bishop Miles's persistent lack of interest, DeMarco kept showing up. He knew, Miles says, that tobacco "should have been an issue that was on my mind. At forty-two, I suffered a heart attack from smoking. I had lost a brother to lung cancer back in 1984 from smoking." When the bishop finally gave DeMarco a hearing, he says, "I'm half listening and half not listening to him, as we are wont to do when we're really just trying to get rid of somebody."

Then DeMarco quoted from an interview by Bob Herbert in the *New York Times* of Sunday, November 28, 1993, in which a former model for Winston cigarettes quoted the response of an R. J. Reynolds executive to his question, "Don't any of you smoke?" "Are you kidding?" came the answer. "We reserve that right for the poor, the young, the black, and the stupid." "My antennae went up," says Miles, "and I immediately sat up and started listening. And that's how I got engaged with Vinny on this campaign and with the whole anti-tobacco movement."

DeMarco wanted the bishop and other faith leaders involved in MCI "because on the gun issue members of the religious community were really activists. They'd pick up the phone—they're the very best at grassroots organizing, mobilizing, action. Pastors can talk to congregations; it's a ready-built network." Faith leadership, and the involvement of the faith community, is critical for four reasons, DeMarco says. First, faith leaders have moral authority: "Just because they are who they are, policymakers have to listen to them. They can't ignore them." If you can mobilize the religious community, "you have the power to get their people to Annapolis. Lawmakers are not comfortable saying no to their religious constituents." Second, the faith community represents "the grassroots; they are where you find people who are going to write the letters and do all the other volunteer work." Third, the media love stories of the faith community versus Big Tobacco: "Good versus Evil—it's classic." And fourth, "faith groups—especially the United Methodists—bring real diversity to the movement: racial, economic, religious, political. Incredible diversity."

In the MCI campaign, ministers—especially ministers with low-income, minority congregations—could also wield their moral authority to dispatch two smokescreens that tobacco lobbyists often lay down to persuade legislators to oppose cigarette tax increases. One is that teenagers today have access to so much money from indulgent parents that raising the price of cigarettes doesn't deter them. The campaign had solid scientific data to refute this deception, a message the Smoke Free Maryland lobbyists were used to delivering effectively to legislators; now the campaign needed the most trusted messengers to deliver that message to the public. The second smokescreen is that tobacco taxes will hurt poor people. DeMarco says he "very rarely" hears that concern voiced by the pastors who actually minister to congregations with poor members. "The African American church leaders kept saying, 'Look, I buried a lot of people who died early from smoking!' White middle- and upper-class liberal pastors were projecting this problem onto poor communities; they were imagining it." When DeMarco went to talk to these leaders, he brought with him one of the reverends who ministered to poor, minority congregations, who made clear that what they were concerned about was not the cost of cigarettes, but their people dying from tobacco addiction.

The United Methodists were natural allies, DeMarco says, because they "had already adopted a resolution on tobacco, so they didn't have to figure out what their position was. Other groups have to go through their bureaucracy and get a vote. Also, ministers and other faith leaders are busy people; it's hard to get their attention. With the religious community, you have to work with their process. You have to go to meetings, conferences—you have to figure out what their process is and work within it." DeMarco had done just that when he had worked with church groups on gun control—and now most of them were open to participating in his excise tax campaign.

The Presbyterians, the Lutherans, and other denominations signed on; the faith leadership organizations actively engaged in the campaign eventually included Clergy United for the Renewal of East Baltimore (CURE), the Interdenominational Ministerial Alliance, the Central Maryland Ecumenical Council, the American Baptist Churches of the South, the United Missionary Baptist Convention, the Maryland Baptist Convention, the American Jewish Congress, the Baltimore Jewish Council, the National Council of Jewish Women, the Church Health Education Resource Union Believers, the Presbytery of Baltimore PC (USA), and the Baltimore-Washington Conference of the United Methodist Church.

How did MCI do it? Board and other staff members of Smoke Free Maryland recruited some of the new signatories to the resolution, but Miles, Schneider, and DeMarco delivered by far the greatest number. Each of the trio brought discrete gifts to the task.

Over many years, Rosanna Miles in her church-based social service and justice advocacy work, along with Bishop Miles, had built trust and confidence throughout a wide network of faith leaders of many denominations. In the course of this work, she and her husband had also come to know well most of Baltimore City's elected officials. Schneider captures the quality of Rosanna Miles's persuasiveness:

> Mrs. Miles is an intuitive, passionate people reader. She does not like public speaking; she doesn't always feel grounded in the science or policy details. Yet she's extremely effective because she talks about the why of our work and the outcomes of our work in a way that hits home with most. She keeps centered on the people we are helping and not the political game that surrounds our work. She can find a personal connection with almost everyone she meets. She's got the most wonderful phone presence. She's always had an ability to talk to the pastors and to other faith community members, which she does expertly, but Rosanna works not only with the faith community, not only with the African American community, but with many, many others.

This is how Miles describes her ability to recruit:

> I draw people in by listening to them and what's going on with them. And that way, I can go ahead and say what I need to say. I never talk to any one group of people the same way because everyone is different. You can't assume that, because you're going to many African American groups, that all of these people are the same. They're not. That's the mistake that many in society make.
>
> So with the coalition, I just feel so compassionate about what we're doing. And I try to relay that. I've talked with politicians who have been totally against what we're doing. And by the time I've finished with them, they'll say, "Ms. Miles, send me the sheet, whatever you need me to sign." If I call someone or write someone a note, and they answer me, I'm going to call them back and thank them. That's how I keep communication open with them.

Rosanna Miles possesses "soft power." DeMarco says he "will never forget when during a crucial vote in the Maryland House of Delegates, one Baltimore City delegate made the mistake of voting against us. After a few phone conversations with Rosanna, the delegate pledged to always be with us in the future, and he has been."

DeMarco would never openly acknowledge that he needed Miles to serve as a gateway to the African American community. She wouldn't let him off the hook:

> I said, "Vinny, every time there's a black meeting with black people, you want me to come. What am I, the token? What do you need me for?"
>
> "I just want you there," he says.
>
> I said, "Vinny, it's all right. They're not going to bother you. It's all right."
>
> And he said, "That's not it." I said, "Yes it is. Because when you go to those other meetings, you don't say, 'Come on, Rosanna, you must go with me.' We went to a meeting for the Collective Banking Group, and there were black pastors who had brought this group together because the banks were not lending money to their people. I'm looking around, I said to Vinny, "Oh, *that's* why you brought me here. It's an African American group."
>
> "That's not it," he insisted.
>
> I said, "Yes it is."

Miles knew, of course, that DeMarco needed her skills in ways that had nothing to do with her color. In time, she would recruit hundreds of organizations—of all races and callings—to sign their campaigns' sometimes serial resolutions. But she couldn't resist teasing DeMarco.

Matching DeMarco's exuberance with his own effervescence, Schneider also proved a uniquely persuasive recruiter. He describes his baptism in reaching out to the faith community as "extremely pleasant," mainly because, he says, DeMarco gave him the confidence to forge ahead on his own. The campaign ran into a snag with the Episcopalians, Schneider says, when "the bishop's health person didn't think a tobacco tax was something they could support: Why should we pick on any one community? Isn't this really going to hurt the poor?" Schneider visited her at her home one Saturday to try to persuade her. "Every time she'd bring up an argument, I'd say, 'You know, it's not really that way. Here's the real truth.' Finally she said, 'I'm going to recommend to the bishop that we sign on.'" Schneider, DeMarco says, has "an uncanny ability to make complex matters understandable to most people. Because he is a terrific listener and respects the people with whom he is talking, he does a great job of really answering the concerns people have about what he is proposing. Schneider could organize a stone."

The Leader

DeMarco was the lead organizer, in part because of the multi-tentacled network he has amassed. Once I saw him distracted by his inability to access instantly a number on his cell phone. He dialed his carrier's service for help. "How many names do you have on your address book?" the service agent asked him. DeMarco had no idea. The agent told him how to retrieve the total—more than eight thousand names. Even if we exclude family members, other morning runners in the park, and bicyclers, DeMarco and Molly Mitchell's huge extended family, school parents, neighbors, and others not involved in DeMarco's advocacy work, his tappable network includes several thousand friends, colleagues, and near strangers who might be useful in some advocacy context.

The closest observers of DeMarco's coalition building over many years offer a compendium of the qualities that enable him to recruit allies to each succeeding campaign, among them enthusiasm, sincerity, intuition, passion, and persuasiveness. "He makes his pitch and you're charged up," says Len Lucchi. In terms of the faith community, specifically, "he recognizes that there are a lot of liberal activists in the state, particularly in the religious community. Every religious denomination has a social justice agenda, and most of the time, we spin our wheels, we do nothing—and I say this as a member of one. Vinny gives those liberal activists who are involved in various causes something to do that's very concrete, very tangible."

"With Vinny," says the Cancer Society's Eric Gally, "you get that incredible feeling that you're doing good for the world; you're about to save somebody's life; you're about to prevent suffering." Similarly, Kathleen Kennedy Townsend, Maryland's lieutenant governor during several of DeMarco's campaigns, notes DeMarco's "extraordinary ability to ask you to be involved and make you want to do it. At least, he makes me want to do it." She calls him "a mythmaker," that is, "he creates a picture about how fabulous you are, tells you you're terrific. You start to believe it. And then you want to be part of his myth, his story, his great adventure. That's what he's terrific at. Of course, all of us know we're really not the type of person that Vinny has created in his mind, but we enjoy the luxury of the story he tells." Lucchi likens DeMarco to "a good trial lawyer": "he knows his audiences. He knows what their emotional trigger points are, and he pushes those buttons."

At the same time, Lucchi says, DeMarco's sincerity comes through, along with his passionate belief in the cause he is advocating. Even pro-tobacco lobbyist Bruce Bereano ekes out praise for DeMarco's energy: "I have never met anybody in this process who had more focus and energy on a single issue than Vinny does. Sometimes that focus and energy carry the day." Lucchi, too, gives credit to DeMarco's can-do persuasiveness: "A lot of people, even activist progressives, will say, 'Oh gee, we can't do that!' They've got ten people telling them it can't be done. Vinny's the guy who's telling them, 'Yes, we can!' And with his track record, he has credibility."

This credibility extends even to the critical—and chronically skeptical—funders. Schneider illustrates:

> We were in a funders meeting, talking about what we had just accomplished, and we came to a point where we said, "Well, we actually don't have money to do this one thing, but if we do eventually get money, we'll do it." Then one of the funders actually said, "Well, how much does that cost?" And Vinny said, "I think it'll cost, like, $35,000." She said, "Well, I'll put in ten. Anybody else match me on that?" Someone else, "I'll put in ten." And we're looking around, saying to ourselves, "Is this happening?" We had no plan of asking them because they'd given so much already. But they all just started to say, "I'll put some cash in there." By the time we left, we had funded that unmet need. And part of that's just simply because we talked to them, and they feel like they are contributing to success, and they're a part of that.

Plainly, behind the endless waves of DeMarco phone calls, e-mails, and smartphone notes lies a high-touch, as well as a high-tech, connection. A fellow organizer with the Campaign for Tobacco-Free Kids, Aaron Doeppers, elaborates: "What Vinny does so well is make personal connections quickly and with almost anyone. This can never be done by e-mail, and while it is an amazing tool that has turbocharged grassroots organizing, I find that all too often people forget its limits. This is not to say Vinny doesn't e-mail—I either receive or am cc'ed a mountain of e-mail from him. But he uses it as an opener or closer in his outreach—he forms his relationships offline where he can talk to someone directly."

Up and Running

By the fall of 1997, the first stage of the campaign was well under way. MCI was up and running, independent of the Smoke Free Maryland Coalition, dedicated solely to enacting the tax increase, then destined to sunset. DeMarco had secured sources of funding beyond the imagination of the coalition leaders. He had brought together strong new allies to help lead the new campaign. And by the end of 1997 he and his team had persuaded more than one hundred citizen organizations across the state to sign the resolution supporting the tax increase (hundreds more would follow). The campaign had gained ground toward constructing the unique political power base that had characterized DeMarco's earlier successes. Delegate Maggie McIntosh, chair of the Maryland House Environmental Matters Committee, who has observed DeMarco in action for many years, captures that uniqueness in words:

He is a master of grassroots organizing in Maryland. He has an idea, and the next thing you know, six months later, he has an office, a budget, and a thousand organizations signed on to help him. The method by which he organizes is intimidating to some legislators. He has cachet when he organizes. There are a lot of lobbyists who come in and say, "All these groups support this cause." And then, as a legislator, I go out and talk to the group leaders and they say, "Yeah, we've signed up, but we don't really care about that."

But not with Vinny. No. The cachet he has with progressive organizations—civic, church, union, labor, civic groups—the trust, the bond that he has to deliver for them on whatever issue that they're working collectively on is so huge that when a legislator gets a communication from Vinny, it's real. It's "Oh, my God, this guy's gone out and organized labor, and my church is on here, and my community group's on here."

It's intimidating to some. It's intimidating because you know that, no matter where you go in your district, or in your church, or in your world, you're going to hear about his campaigns on behalf of the children and families of Maryland.

The MCI coalition was growing, but it was not yet "intimidating" enough in McIntosh's sense of the term. That would begin to be true only as DeMarco unleashed the campaign tool that complemented his outsized organizing: media advocacy.

3

Media Advocacy:
"A Giant Telephone"

The unwillingness of the 1997 Maryland legislature to raise the cigarette tax was not the result of the legislators' rejection of Smoke Free Maryland's arguments. The legislators simply weren't listening to them. They weren't listening because *they didn't have to listen.* They didn't have to listen because their constituents weren't demanding that they listen. The coalition might have produced a panel of Nobel Prize–winning scientists to testify on the proven connection between high taxes and falling cigarette consumption, and the outcome would have been no different—as long as legislative indifference brought no political consequences.

DeMarco's task was to make sure that this time the legislators would learn that *they had to listen.* Neither authoritative testimony nor persuasive lobbying would teach them that; only aroused and mobilized voters would. Because DeMarco views the media "as a giant telephone which I can use to talk with the people of Maryland," he would begin the public stages of the campaign by blitzing the mass media and would not let up for two years. Free, earned mass media coverage, with a tactical sprinkling of timely paid advertising, would be DeMarco's antidote to the invisible influence of the tobacco lobby.

DeMarco's forays into the media were launched simultaneously with stages 1 and 2, initial organizing and recruiting signatories to the campaign resolution. Well before he would seriously seek legislative action, these public education initiatives would carry embedded advocacy messages in addition to the core *public health* message, which was the connection between high taxes and low teenage use of tobacco. These messages would convey the political safety of supporting tobacco tax increases and, even more important, the political risks of failing to do so. The primary targets of these messages would be the legislators who had felt no need to pay attention in 1997, and who it was DeMarco's job to ensure would end up paying very close attention in the future. Thus his media advocacy would sharpen its focus on the elected power holders and increase its intensity after the initial organizing stages.

This media advocacy strategy was central to DeMarco's campaign plan from the outset:

> I like to have an overview in my head of the series of events I want to do over the course of the campaign to get our message out. You want to make sure every event is newsworthy, but you also don't want to wear out your welcome with the reporters. Also it is important to recognize that a major paper like the *Baltimore Sun* has different bureaus and reporters—business, political, faith, and so on—who might be interested in different events. For the Maryland Children's Initiative, I early on figured we would try to do several key events, including releasing poll results; announcing the formation of the coalition and the endorsement of key groups like the faith leaders and the students; launching the voter education campaign and ballyhooing its results; announcing our radio ads and other paid media; and getting coverage of events in Annapolis, like a rally. Though we needed to be ready to take advantage of other great media opportunities as they came up, having this plan in my mind helped a great deal.
>
> For each event, such as the release of the poll, the first step was to frame the event in a way that would attract media attention. Something like "Marylanders support tobacco taxes." Second, we had people as messengers in whom the media would be interested, like nationally renowned pollsters. Third, we would put together a short and effective media advisory that highlighted our message and attractive messengers.

Edging Closer to Political Action

Philanthropies have become increasingly wary of the IRS prohibition against using tax-exempt dollars for political advocacy or lobbying, especially when such funding results in unwelcome media attention. DeMarco knows this well, which is why he is beyond scrupulous in following the rules. Throughout all his campaigns, DeMarco kept in frequent contact with his legal advisor, Michael Pretl, one of Maryland's premier experts on nonprofit legal issues. With Pretl's guidance, DeMarco faithfully complies with the complex IRS rules regarding the use and reporting of expenditures for polling, advertising, and other media activities. From the very beginning, MCI accounted carefully for funds applied to these activities in three relevant categories: pure public education, grassroots lobbying, and general lobbying. Funds from a separate advocacy organization were employed for any activities related to election politics. Yet, within the confines imposed by the IRS rules, the campaign was able, as Schneider says, "to create an environment for policy change to occur." The messages were primarily targeted to the general public, but also—as in an echo chamber—they would be heard by the legislators. The public education had multiple objectives:

> Raise the awareness of the people of Maryland concerning the health and social hazards of cigarette smoking, especially teenage smoking
>
> Educate Marylanders about the effectiveness of very high cigarette taxes in diverting teenagers from a lifelong addiction
>
> Educate Marylanders on the benefits that would flow to causes dear to many citizens from the revenues generated by new cigarette tax increases
>
> Counteract the scientific disinformation that tobacco company propagandists were disseminating to cloud the public mind on the health benefits of cigarette tax increases
>
> Educate journalists on the merits of tobacco tax increases so that they, in turn, could educate their readers
>
> Appeal to the pride of Marylanders to support the largest cigarette tax increase in the nation
>
> Publicize the phenomenal growth of the MCI in a way that inspired organizations to leap aboard the campaign bandwagon
>
> Redirect the media's boredom with the tobacco tax issue as a nonstarter in Annapolis to a growing awareness that a powerful popular movement was brewing
>
> Raise the profile of cigarette tax increase demands on the agenda of the next, and the next, Maryland legislative sessions
>
> Persuade Maryland's elected officials that, in voters' minds, this tax was different from all others—it was popular, even a $1.50 increase
>
> Serve notice on Maryland legislators and would-be legislators that this movement could motivate a significant shift of Election Day votes against legislators who continued to vote for Big Tobacco
>
> Impress upon legislators who ignored this movement that they should beware its political benefits for those who might challenge them in party primaries or the general election

Though DeMarco's plan was to stay away from lobbying until after the 1998 elections, the lawmakers were in his sights from the onset.

Designing Hooks and Messages

The first task for a media advocate is to get—and sustain—the interest of journalists and editors, the gatekeepers to the media. Though the ostensible subject of DeMarco's media initiatives was health, for his objective—reaching legislators—this meant reaching political reporters more than health reporters. He would need to generate stories, first, with news "hooks" or "pegs" that grabbed political reporters' attention, and second, with messages aimed at legislators as well as the general public.

DeMarco's initial tactics in creating newsworthy stories and delivering the desired messages, the dual objectives of media advocacy, illustrate his resourcefulness. He knew that, carefully packaged, polls serve these dual objectives: reporters, political reporters especially, never seem to tire of poll-based stories. The October 23 *Baltimore Sun* story by Scott Shane ran a two-column headline—"Across Party Lines, Voters Favor Raising Cigarette Tax by $1.50"—that landed above the fold on the front page. The article led with, "Anti-smoking activists will push for a whopping $1.50-a-pack cigarette tax next year, and they warn that lawmakers who oppose them will be displeasing voters." The story hammered home this point through the reportage on the presence of the pollster Celinda Lake: "'These numbers are startling,' said Lake, a nationally prominent pollster who has worked mainly for Democrats. 'Being willing to change your vote over an issue like this is very unusual.'" Shane also quoted several participants in the news conferences, the first a Maryland legislator: "We now know clearly where the majority of Marylanders stand," said state delegate Elizabeth Bobo. "It's an eye-opener for any legislators who freeze up when they hear the word 'tax.'"

The campaign squeezed more educational juice from the poll in its third release of results to the media. A story by Tom Stuckey, the Annapolis-based Associated Press (AP) political writer, ran prominently in several local daily and weekly papers (and on *USA Today*'s state news page) on November 23 and featured the announcement by "a group of anti-smoking lawmakers" that they would introduce the $1.50-per-pack tax increase in the next session of the legislature. But its main content was a reprise of the poll results. The anti-smoking lawmakers, Stuckey reported, had been "buoyed by the poll," and he proceeded to spell out its main findings. The message: wavering legislators take note—cigarette tax increases are good politics.

A second message embedded in the Stuckey story was designed for yet another key audience: the leadership of advocacy groups with goals different from those of Smoke Free Maryland's members. The appeal to them was that the cigarette tax proceeds would finance programs they and their members cherished. It also sent a message to the state's tobacco farmers, diminishing in number but still politically potent, that could soften their opposition: "To win more support this time, [the lawmakers] plan to use the new tax revenues for an anti-smoking public relations campaign; school aid; treatment programs for addiction to drugs, alcohol, and tobacco; and a program to help tobacco farmers switch to other crops." The article closed by quoting a call to arms by Smoke Free Maryland president Joseph Adams: "If the people lead, their leaders in the legislature eventually will follow."

Cultivating Media Relationships

The media's willingness, reflected in news accounts of the poll release, to repeatedly report on what would seem to be the same story leaves Glenn Schneider marveling: "I always found it amazing that Vinny could repackage something that we'd done five times already and still get media to come out time after time and cover it."

This consistent media response is no accident. "First," says DeMarco, "I work very hard on finding out who the reporters are in all the media who would cover our initiative and getting to know them. My twin goals are to build a relationship and to educate them about the issue. Like with the coalition, I think it is very important to build these relationships before you are calling them to cover an event." He sustains these relationships over time. Every few weeks for many years, for example, DeMarco has met for breakfast with the *Sun*'s senior political columnist, Fraser Smith, trading Maryland political intelligence and gossip, whether or not he has a story to sell.

Whenever DeMarco schedules an event, he is on top of the reporters from before the event takes place to its follow-up: "Part of this is writing a good press release which has good quotes, particularly for reporters who can't make it to the event. Finally, and this is an important lesson I learned from Bernie Horn, I call the reporters late in the day after they have had a chance to talk with the other side so that I can answer any statements the other side made and make my case once again for the story I want."

Another Media Hook:
The Campaign Launch (Again and Again)

Next in the 1997 cigarette excise tax effort came a press release announcing the December 23 unveiling of MCI itself, with a press conference, at which the media would witness "prominent Maryland organizations launch a statewide initiative calling for a $1.50 increase in the state cigarette tax to reduce teen smoking and fund pro-child programs. The organizations will sign a resolution endorsing the initiative and pledge to have 100 organizations from across Maryland sign the resolution by January 14, 1998, the first day of the 1998 General Assembly Session."

The peg on which reporters could hang their stories was the formation and launching of MCI, a cigarette tax campaign with, the press release promised, "non-traditional partners." The story would be framed as a demonstration of the broad appeal of the campaign, an incentive for as yet uncommitted organizations not to be left behind a popular train already working up a good head of steam, and a message to legislators that a trainload of potent advocacy groups would soon be at their doors.

At the press conference, Smoke Free Maryland's Joseph Adams hailed "the first time in the nation that a $1.50 cigarette tax is being seriously proposed at the state level, and the first time in Maryland that such powerful and important organizations have come together to make this a priority issue." Adams read an enthusiastic letter from former U.S. surgeon general C. Everett Koop, who endorsed the initiative and appealed to Marylanders' pride: their state could be the first "to seriously consider the kind of cigarette tax increase which will really make a difference in reducing teen smoking." Each lead organization was represented by its leader, and each got the organization's tailored educational messages out.

The *Baltimore Sun* and other Maryland papers again paid attention, again on their front pages. These stories illustrate an observation of the *Sun's* Fraser Smith that "Vinny is not a first-paragraph guy," quoting the organization leader, then the authority figures, then the poll results, and deep in the body of the story, DeMarco, "president of the initiative group." As in almost every campaign-generated story, DeMarco's words succinctly framed a key message to lawmakers, in this case: "Vinny DeMarco . . . said that if the General Assembly does not pass such a tax increase during the 90-day session that begins in January, his organization will make it a major issue in November's election."

Though often not subtle, DeMarco is so on target and clear when he speaks to journalists that it is his words that seize the attention of the headline writer or the editor who chooses what quotations to highlight in a sidebar—such as this typically pithy and straightforward quotation from DeMarco that a local paper inset in boldface type: "What the legislature of Maryland will see is that the people of Maryland want this to happen."

Paid Media Advocacy

At this critical juncture in the campaign, as in others to come, the DeMarco team turned to paid media advocacy to shore up public support for the tax, and to help reframe journalists' perspectives. For example, to help dispel the troublesome revelation in the poll by Celinda Lake that only a bare majority of voters understood that higher cigarette taxes meant less teen smoking, Bernie Horn and Len Lucchi developed a radio ad featuring Lieutenant Governor Townsend that was sponsored by the medically authoritative Maryland Medical Society:

> Hi, I'm Kathleen Kennedy Townsend, lieutenant governor of Maryland. I'm also the mother of four school-aged daughters. Like all parents, I want my children to grow up happy and healthy . . . So I'm very concerned about teen smoking. Right now, smoking among teenagers is on the rise in Maryland. More Maryland children alive today will die from smoking than from any other single cause. That's 85,000 of our children victimized by tobacco.
> How can we protect our children? Public health experts say the best way is to increase the price of cigarettes. They've proven that, when the price of tobacco goes up, teen smoking goes down. And the higher we increase the price, the more kids we save. The big tobacco companies don't like it, but it's the right thing to do for all of our children.

The Horn and Lucchi team also created a powerful print ad to dramatize the extent of the risk of smoking to teenagers. Sponsored by MCI, it displayed sixty appealing Maryland kids, with the letter *X* marked through twenty of their faces. "Today, 60 Maryland children will become cigarette addicts," headlined the ad. Then, below the portraits: "20 of them will die before their time."

Neither ad addressed legislators; neither qualified as lobbying. But legislators and other policymakers saw and heard the ads—a bonus. So did some voters and, more important, so did most of the reporters covering the tax issue.

To get the attention of African American legislators, some of whom had been wooed successfully by tobacco lobbyists to offer support, and to assuage the anxieties of liberals and liberal churches that resisted signing the resolution out of concern for the effect of the tax on poor people, Horn and Lucchi produced this radio ad featuring the morally authoritative Bishop Miles:

> This is the Reverend Douglas Miles. For years tobacco companies have been targeting our teens. Working to addict our children to their deadly drug.

Big Tobacco has put billboards all over our neighborhoods. Given away free samples to get our children hooked. And kept their prices low to keep us addicted to cigarettes. Working together we stood up to Big Tobacco and won the fight to get their billboards out of our neighborhoods.

But we must do more.

Raising cigarette prices will cut teen smoking. And is one of the best things we can do to protect our health. Now Big Tobacco is trying to convince us that higher cigarette prices would hurt poor people.

Don't be fooled.

The only people that higher cigarette prices will hurt are the tobacco companies trying to addict our families. God has given us all the gift of life. And we must do our part, by keeping our children safe and well.

Press Hound?

Nothing maddens tobacco lobbyist Bruce Bereano more than DeMarco's prowess at gaining media attention. In Bereano's view, DeMarco's press attention "is all about him. He's egotistical, self-centered. He stands up there and spins it and says, 'You know, I won this!'" Bereano is not alone. Even some advocates on DeMarco's side of the issues feel this way. Bernie Horn acknowledges that "a lot of people in Maryland dislike Vinny because they think he's a press hound—and being a press hound is something that definitely pisses off the non–press hounds, whether you're a press-hound legislator or a press-hound lobbyist."

No one would accuse DeMarco of being media shy. He delights in media coverage that advances his campaigns, but there's little evidence that he pursues it to promote himself. As Horn concludes: "There's a certain amount of jealousy, but also, there's a lot of misunderstanding. You have to get all this press; that's the whole idea. You cannot pass one of these bills without getting the press. Vinny gets this reputation because he's very effective."

Yet this was only the beginning of the campaign's media advocacy (and only a sampling of its ubiquitous presence). At each of the remaining stages of the campaign, DeMarco would continue his pursuit of media coverage, framing the media messages to directly and indirectly target legislators and their leaders.

4

The 1998 State Elections: Bridgehead for Action

So extensive and favorable were the results of the MCI launch in December that many committed legislators and advocates, along with DeMarco's deputy Glenn Schneider, began to harbor hopes that they were going to pass a big cigarette tax in 1998. "Had a big argument with people," DeMarco says. "They asked, 'Why is this a two-year plan? Let's just get it done this year.'" While he agreed with Schneider that they should give it their best shot—"You just don't ever know what can happen," Schneider said—DeMarco was certain it would take two years from the launch of the campaign in the summer of 1997, as well as an election, for the public education and coalition-building stages of the initiative to build sufficient political steam to win.

DeMarco had a long list of good reasons for his certainty. At this juncture, the campaign was not a threat even to wavering legislators. Mike Miller, still Senate president, still with virtual control over the Senate, remained adamant in his opposition. Miller's legislative allies—senior senators from tobacco-growing districts—still sat on the key Senate committees. Most Republican delegates and senators were still riding the "No tax increase—read my lips" crusade (immortalized by the Senior Bush's presidential campaign pledge). Even Democrats were skeptical of MCI's polls showing voter support for a cigarette tax increase. Finally, Governor Glendening was gun-shy of another embarrassing defeat at the hands of the legislature. Though a committed tobacco tax advocate, he was looking over his shoulder at the last election's close call; his Republican opponent then, Ellen Sauerbrey, had never ceased running and gearing up for a November 1998 rematch. Her mantra? Tax cuts.

Stage 3. The Trial Run

Despite all of these unpromising conditions, DeMarco supported an all-out effort to force the legislature to confront the tax issue in the 1998 session, which would open in early January. His goals remained the same: "to set the agenda, to get it before the public. Put the bill in, hold a lot of major press conferences, get hearings where we laid out our proposal, hear what the other side had to say, hear what the questions were."

> One of the most important things in this kind of strategy is to understand when you're not going to pass something. It's a whole different way of dealing with the legislature when you know that they're not going to pass it. You're working to raise public consciousness. That's controversial with some advocates who say you have to work to pass it every single year because every time you don't pass it more kids are dying, but my response is: "It's not going to pass. You can do all these things to get it passed, but it won't. But you're not going to pass it next year either if you don't deal with it as part of a long-term strategy."
>
> There's a lot less tension in your stomach at a hearing where you don't think your bill's going to pass than at a hearing where you really need to pass the bill. It's very useful to have the attacks against the bill when you have time to adjust it. You learn why it didn't pass and you can respond.

Media Advocacy for the Trial Run

As the 1998 legislative session approached, DeMarco's cultivation of the media began to pay off in a second wave of media coverage and framing, this time with a salvo of strong editorials. Early on, DeMarco says, "We spent a good deal of time meeting with and educating editorial board writers. It is very important to take time to reach out to the ed board writers and answer their questions long before you ask them to write an editorial."

On November 16, 1997, a *Baltimore Sun* editorial called upon Governor Glendening to ignore the General Assembly's defeat of anti-smoking measures he had backed the previous year and "give it a second try, especially if the proceeds are earmarked for programs aimed at reducing youth smoking." Why should Glendening butt his head against the legislative wall again? Because not only did the Lake poll show overwhelming support for a "whopping" tax, editorialized the *Sun*, but "equally telling were poll results indicating voters would desert incumbents who oppose higher cigarette taxes aimed at cutting teen smoking. This is especially true of Democratic women, Democrats under 45, and Democrats who are African American. By overwhelming numbers they say they would vote for a Republican over a Democrat incumbent who supported the tobacco industry's position."

As Maryland's legislators were arriving in town for the 1998 session, the Annapolis *Capital* headlined its December 26 editorial, "Cigarette Tax Hike Would Be Healthy for Pols, Kids." Apart from their inclusion of snippets of tobacco lobby rhetoric, these articles and editorials not only gave full-blown coverage to the campaign's relaunch, but also framed the issues exactly as DeMarco had hoped.

Meanwhile, DeMarco and Schneider and their core team would walk a tightrope, as Schneider explains: "You can't tell anybody that you are trying to push for a bill they care deeply about that you don't expect to win. You can call it a trial run later, but not when you're fighting for it." The first MCI event in 1998—and the first news peg—was the introduction early in the session of the $1.50 tax increase bill in the Senate and in the House by DeMarco's inside legislative leaders, House Ways and Means Committee chair Sheila Hixson and Senate Budget and Taxation Committee member Chris Van Hollen— both forceful and influential advocates. This coincided with an announcement from MCI that the bill was now backed by a coalition of "more than 150 organizations."

The media coverage during the session proved at least as broad and felicitously framed as before, recycling many facts and quotations from earlier stories. And DeMarco was already signaling the campaign's election strategy by unleashing a threat that the February 15 Easton *Star-Democrat* ran as a banner alongside its story: "We are going to make sure every voter in Maryland knows how his candidate voted on this issue." Nonetheless, the political columnists remained as skeptical as DeMarco about the bill's chances, although the *Baltimore Sun*'s Fraser Smith on February 10, 1998, dutifully reported the game assertion of the bill's Senate sponsor, Chris Van Hollen, that this year would be a different story: "We recognize that we have an uphill battle. But one thing has changed. [Tobacco] company documents show that they clearly targeted teen-agers. That has made people's blood boil." Then Smith's skepticism resurfaced: "But, the tobacco interests will surely ask, how much boiling will go on in the blood of those who smoke now—25% of all Marylanders. They claim their lobbyists are prepared to marshal all the usual arguments. The tax will drive customers into neighboring states, hurt Maryland farmers, and impose an unfair duty on a legal product."

Smith and DeMarco proved prescient. Nonsmokers' blood may have simmered, but it did not boil. On March 25, the Senate Budget and Taxation Committee rejected even a scaled-down version of the tax increase, killing it for the 1998 session.

The Payoffs

To the casual observer, the MCI campaign had gone nowhere during the 1998 session. Not true. The advocates this time were not sucker-punched. They had educated the committee that would later decide the fate of the tax increase bill. They had found out who on that committee was ready to vote for it, and who was not. The effort energized the coalition, which was exuberantly represented in committee hearings through a diversity of strong witnesses and hundreds of attending activists. The hearings also provided a test of the effectiveness of the arguments and spokespeople testifying for the tax increase—and teased out the identities and arguments of the bill's opponents.

DeMarco cites another insight gleaned from the trial run, which would force a major change in the campaign's legislative strategy for the 1999 session: the chair of the Senate Budget and Taxation Committee, Barbara Hoffman, would oppose any bill that allocated tax revenue. This was hardly good news, but it was critical intelligence. Gaining Hoffman's support was a make-or-break condition for getting the tax bill passed in the Senate. She strongly supported a naked tax increase—"would have supported a five-dollar increase," DeMarco judged. But as the chair of a powerful committee that determines how tax moneys are both raised and allocated, she despised the practice of legislative "hypothecation"—allocating tax revenues by permanent law, not by the normal process of annual budgeting that was the Budget and Taxation Committee's domain. The state Senate led by President Miller would remain a hard sell, even with Hoffman's support. DeMarco met with Hoffman shortly after the 1998 session closed. She would not budge. "Oh, man, Barbara," he thought, "even after all my kowtowing." But the coalition would, sooner or later, need to meet her objections.

As the session closed, *Sun* columnist Michael Olesker turned the legislators' education decibel level up a notch, targeting Hoffman and "those sellouts on the Maryland Senate's Budget and Taxation Committee." With outrage that would fuel the November elections, Olesker enumerated the tobacco companies' every corrupt and crooked act that the media had exposed, demanding: "What's that make members of the Budget and Taxation Committee? Accessories after the fact, which ought to carry its own penalties. At the voting booth, at least."

Stage 4. The Candidate Pledge Campaign

The trial run in the 1998 legislative session, as planned, set the stage for the coming September primary and November general elections. DeMarco was clear: the elections of 1998—not anything the campaign did or said after the elections—would determine whether a tax bill would pass during the 1999 legislative session. In the spring and early summer of 1998, the campaign would focus squarely on two target audiences: voters and legislators. It would use the election cycle, first, to persuade all candidates for the legislature or statewide office to sign a pledge to endorse the tobacco tax increase, and, second, to educate the public about which candidates supported the tobacco tax and which did not.

Since the tax increase never came out of committee in the 1998 legislative session, the vast majority of legislators never had to vote on it. To DeMarco's way of thinking, the only way to let voters know how incumbents and challengers stood on the issue was to ask them to sign the pledge, and to tell the voters who signed and who refused to sign.

The voter campaign would be strictly nonpartisan. MCI would never endorse candidates, pledge signers or not. And the schedule was tight. "July and August of 1998 was when we would win—or not win—this campaign," DeMarco says. "If you're asking a legislator to do something during a session, you're just another lobbyist, another pain in the neck. At election time, if they're in a tight race especially, you're somebody they've got to pay attention to."

Kids, Polls, and God: More Earned Media

No sooner had the Senate Budget and Taxation Committee killed the tax bill in March 1998 than DeMarco's media advocacy shifted its focus to the fall elections. The MCI team was out again to every corner of the state, no matter how few its voters, organizing local meetings, public forums, and press events. Each featured as speakers not only local civic and political leaders and health and children's advocates, but also young people.

A typical story—one of dozens of similar articles—ran on April 10, 1998, in the Easton *Star-Democrat* on Maryland's rural eastern shore. Under the four-column banner headline "Local Organizations Campaign to Raise Tobacco Tax over Next Three Years" appeared a three-column photo of students holding the MCI banner. Talbot County readers learned that 25 of the 225 organizations now endorsing MCI were from Talbot County and heard the concerns of Kami Burns, an eighth grader at Easton Middle School and a member of the No Ands, Ifs, or Butts Club. Kami, who voiced her disappointment with anti-tax legislators because many of her classmates "use tobacco every day," suggested that those legislators "deserve an 'F'" for performance. Now MCI churned out news of a new poll, a new campaign launch, a new press release, a new press conference—eliciting a front-page, section B, above-the-fold *Baltimore Sun* article headlined, on July 3, 1998, "Smoking Foes See Election Issue." In the second paragraph, DeMarco, speaking now on behalf of 286 allied organizations, says: "We'll be launching a major campaign to make sure Maryland voters know how candidates stand on this issue."

The pledge MCI would ask every candidate to sign distilled the legislative essence of the broad resolution that MCI coalition members had signed as they joined. It would allow signers no wiggle room after the elections but would tie them tightly to support for the $1.50 tax increase. As a first step, the campaign sent formal letters asking each candidate to sign the pledge. After that, "ask" became an understatement—"pressure" or even "hound" would be more accurate. Coalition members in each electoral district would call, write, and lie in wait either at candidate forums or at the candidate's office.

Simultaneously, media coverage of the new poll was hammering home its conclusion that even Republican voters supported the bill: 58 percent in favor to 30 percent opposed. DeMarco had calculated that results from a new poll would accomplish a number of short-term goals. They would (1) offer fresh evidence of the political potency of the cigarette tax bill among Maryland voters in the next elections; (2) strengthen the credibility of this message to candidates, because of the highly respected joint Democratic/Republican polling team, led by Robert Green of Penn, Schoen and Berland Associates, President Clinton's pollsters; (3) allow the campaign to localize the poll's findings to each political region of the state; (4) generate a new round of media public education; and, not least, (5) reinforce the support of the hard-money donors by demonstrating anew that the cigarette tax increase was an election-winning issue.

The July 3 *Baltimore Sun* article quoted the pollsters themselves: "'It is abundantly clear that, for Republicans to be competitive, candidates have to be responsive to the very broad concern expressed in this poll about teen smoking,' said [Republican pollster Steven] Wagner, who, in 1994, had conducted much of the research that powered the GOP's 'Contract with America.'"

DeMarco and Schneider doggedly continued to generate—or piggyback on—story after story, forever finding or refurbishing a new media hook:

June 30, *Baltimore Sun*: "Foes of Smoking Take Heart as Politicians Quit Puffing" quotes DeMarco.

July 2, *Cumberland Times-News*: "Group Targets Teen Smoking" quotes DeMarco.

July 9, Howard County *Columbia Flier*: "Breathtaking Trend" (young blacks smoking more) quotes Schneider.

July 17, Montgomery County *Gazette*: "Cigarette Tax to Fund Prevention" quotes DeMarco.

In mid-July, as the primary campaigns began to get attention, MCI un-leashed its most powerful weapon: the clerics. The news peg was the breadth of support for the tax increase. On Monday, July 13, 1998, representatives of al-most all the members of the Central Maryland Ecumenical Council appeared at a press conference. The next day, a *Sun* headline read: "Clerics Back Md. Tobacco Tax Increase; Coalition Supports $1.50-per-Pack Rise Aimed at Teen Agers; 'Nobody Should Smoke'; Denominations' Decision Termed 'a Break-through.'" As Glenn Schneider remarks gleefully: "When the story aired on local TV, one station had the story pegged as 'God vs. Tobacco.' You can't get any better than that!"

The *Sun* also quoted a new media-worthy spokesman, the veteran national tobacco control advocate and Boston law professor Richard Daynard. Until the Central Maryland Ecumenical Council announced its support, Daynard said, "as far as he is aware, the involvement of the religious groups in the anti-tobacco movement has been limited to resolutions passed in annual conven-tions and the divestment of tobacco stock by many denominations." Buried deep in the story, as DeMarco had intended, his own quotation tied the cler-ics' commitment firmly to their determination to hold legislative candidates accountable for supporting or opposing the $1.50 tobacco tax increase.

While the grassroots activists were pressuring the candidates in person, the media advocacy was constantly reminding them of the benefits and risks of signing—or not signing—the pledge.

The Mother's Milk of Politics

As the campaign moved on from what MCI legal advisor Mike Pretl had demonstrated to funders was permissible "public education" (even when we have here labeled it "media advocacy") to directly educating voters about the pledge signers, DeMarco and Schneider would need political education funds, or hard money.

Pretl had been the legal advisor for all of DeMarco's gun control work and was one of Maryland's most expert public interest lawyers. For MCI, he had set up a dual legal structure: first, a nonprofit, tax-exempt organization, formally known by its IRS tax designation as a 501(c)(3), to which founda-tions and other philanthropic donors could safely contribute tax-exempt dol-lars. Pretl made sure that this entity secured the so-called IRS "h" designation that allowed it to spend up to 20 percent of its total expenditures on lobby-ing. Second, they created a parallel IRS recognized 501(c)(4) entity that could lobby and influence elections with much fewer restrictions but could not raise tax-deductible contributions. Pretl's counsel on how to structure the finan-cial operations of the two groups, DeMarco says, kept him "out of jail." Each group—whose personnel were the same—had its own board, and Pretl served as counsel on both. The boards included representatives of the key organizations that made MCI work, such as faith leaders, children's groups, and the teachers' union, all of whom now trusted DeMarco's leadership. He was the executive director of both organizations. The staff and DeMarco would scrupulously allocate their time between the two, and DeMarco would make sure that the 501(c)(4) money would pay for time spent on lobbying and electoral activity that the 501(c)(3) could not.

Some of this non-tax-deductible money came from one of the key MCI coalition partners, the Maryland State Teachers Association, whose interest lay not only in reducing kids' smoking, but also in the revenue that would go to children's issues such as education. DeMarco reached out to partners for whom a major priority was less increasing the tobacco tax than it was electing the candidates (mostly Democrats) who were most likely to support the partners' other interests—interests that might appeal less to the public than the cigarette tax now appeared to. Among these were DeMarco's friends in the labor movement, particularly the state employees' union, who feared the anti-union thrust of many Republicans and some conservative Democrats. Another funding source DeMarco explored were his friends among the state trial lawyers, who worried that the tort reform agenda of the Republicans would shield corporate wrongdoers from the reach of consumer class-action lawsuits. MCI's polling numbers convinced these groups that supporting tobacco tax increases would help elect the candidates they favored. They saw the light—and they came up with the money.

Getting the Number One Signature

Among the first signatories to the pledge had to be Governor Glendening, whose wholehearted support and signature would signal Democratic candidates to jump aboard and whose unequivocal leadership in the next legislative session would be crucial to winning. Getting that signature proved more challenging than DeMarco had anticipated. Yes, Glendening had introduced the thirty-six-cent tax. Yes, both his parents had died of smoking-induced cancer. "Personally," says DeMarco, "he's 100 percent for this. But like any governor, he's got advisors on all sides, and he hears the good, the bad, and the ugly." The "ugly" was coming from Glendening's top political advisors in the form of a scenario for the 1998 election in which Republican candidate Ellen Sauerbrey would hang Glendening on a cross of tax profligacy if he signed the pledge. She had come close in 1994. With a potent issue, she could win in 1998.

DeMarco decided on a dramatic public strategy to pressure Glendening and all the other gubernatorial candidates into signing the pledge. He sent each of them a pledge form and a letter that asked them to sign it by May 31, 1998, World No Tobacco Day. On that day, he informed them, student leaders were going to hold a public rally in Baltimore harbor where—Boston Tea Party style—they would declare their independence from tobacco and announce which candidates for governor had endorsed MCI. The implication, of course, was that those who didn't sign would be metaphorically tossed into the harbor. Next, DeMarco and his team asked the by now 367 coalition partners to contact the candidates and demand that they sign the pledge. This was the first time the partners were mobilized, and they responded eagerly and vigorously.

When DeMarco visited with Sauerbrey, one of the two Republican candidates for governor, she dismissed tobacco addiction as akin to her own "addiction" to chocolate. She stuck with her anti-tobacco-tax stance, later announcing: "I have no intention of raising taxes. Period. The purpose of taxation is to raise revenue, not change behavior." Neither Republican candidate signed the pledge. In the Democrats' camp, as the Baltimore harbor tobacco rally grew closer, both of Glendening's primary opponents continued to hear from voters, and both signed.

DeMarco often taps his dense network of allies to find exactly the right person to speak to a wavering or unhappy power holder. When he was pressuring Governor Glendening to sign the campaign pledge to support the cigarette tax increase, he says: "I sent letters to him, contacted everybody I knew in the governor's office, sending them copies of the poll. Peter Hamm, his communications director, was our biggest advocate. I met with people on the campaign staff often, talked with them a lot about why the governor should sign the pledge."

The morning of the harbor rally, DeMarco got a call from the governor's office staff: Glendening would be very supportive, but he was not going to sign the pledge. MCI's press conference was scheduled for two o'clock. "My stomach was in knots," DeMarco says. "I did not want to say we didn't have Parris Glendening signed on. I called a couple of people on the staff and argued with them that not signing was a big mistake." At noon, a call came from the Glendening campaign headquarters: the governor would sign. DeMarco's allies on the inside of Glendening's campaign, abetted by the media-generated pressure and Glendening's own apolitical commitment to tobacco control, had won the day.

The harbor rally was a rousing event—and roused great press for the formal launch of MCI's voter education campaign, though it had informally been under way for months. The AP's State House reporter Tom Stuckey sent out a story on the AP Maryland wire with the intended message: "As political campaigns nationwide reverberate with calls for tax cuts, two Maryland gubernatorial candidates are openly advocating a tax increase. That does not mean that Gov. Parris Glendening and Democratic challenger Eileen Rehrmann have taken leave of their senses—an increase in the levy on cigarettes is a popular one with many voters."

That Glendening's staff had merely pledged that the governor would sign became an issue over the next three weeks. DeMarco called the governor's campaign office every day in his personal effort to get the promised signature. Then, he found the right messenger—the head of the teachers' union, Michael Butera, who he knew was very close to the governor. Butera simply told the governor, "Would you *give* Vinny the paper!" The governor finally came through, and now DeMarco had even more leverage to get other candidates to sign.

Educating the Other Five Hundred Candidates

Right after the early July filing deadline for candidates for the General Assembly, MCI had sent a pledge form and letter to every person who had filed for one of the 188 electoral seats—more than five hundred candidates. The deadline for returning the pledge was August 24, the letter informed them. After that date, MCI would widely publicize who had signed on and who had not.

Like Glendening, some candidates who supported the tax increase were at first reluctant to sign the pledge. Legislators don't like to be hemmed in, though many of them, along with Glendening, had signed a pledge from DeMarco four years before on the gun control issue. DeMarco & Co. waited a courteous two weeks, then phoned and called upon every candidate who had supported the increase in the past. "I did a lot of driving to people's offices to put it in front of them," DeMarco says. "I spent a lot of time with people I knew." Many candidates were simply not sure how they stood on the tax increase. What they did know was that they preferred to wait and see which way the political winds blew. Others had no intention of supporting the tax—at least until a credible opponent had signed the pledge and made an issue of it. DeMarco's strategy here was clear: "We of course ignored candidates we knew would be against us. You go for the swing people whom you need to pressure."

It was at this point that the coalition hit the road, with members traveling all over the state to campaign events, where they told candidates, DeMarco said: "'I want you to sign that pledge.' People would have community forums and someone would say, 'Did you sign that Children's Initiative pledge yet?'" The unique strength of this strategy was that it was precisely in each state legislative district that the coalition's allied organizations were at home, literally but also figuratively, at ease in approaching local candidates. In every district there were churches whose leaders were active in the MCI campaign. There were organized teachers; there were active student groups; there were friends and family members of candidates who learned about the pledge from pulpits and from organization newsletters; there were voters who didn't belong to any group but had been energized by the barrage of media stories. Orchestrating all this there were DeMarco and MCI staffers Rosanna Miles and Linda Coveleskie on the phones all day, or showing up at candidates' events, invited or not. Meanwhile, Glenn Schneider, who was funded with 501(c)(3) money—not to be used for political campaigning—capitalized on the heightened news coverage to recruit new member groups for the MCI coalition.

As the pledge became a topic of election campaigns, candidates heard about it, DeMarco says, "not just from us but from people who were important to them." He still marvels. "It was one of the most amazing things I've ever seen happen—where people who you never thought would sign on signed on because they were getting a lot of pressure, especially people in tight races." For example, regarding a key signer, Senate Majority Leader Clarence Blount, DeMarco explains: "At this point, it's massive pressure, but it's individualized. We found people in the city who were close to him and they got him to sign."

Prince Georges County senator Gloria Lawlah was one of the most critical targets because she was a potential swing vote on the Senate Budget and Taxation Committee. She did not want to sign the pledge. She wasn't sure how she felt about raising cigarette taxes, but she was sure she didn't want to offend Senate President Mike Miller, who had given her a seat on that powerful committee. Lawlah was locked in a tough primary race against the Reverend C. Anthony Muse, a United Methodist minister who not only signed the pledge, but also was vocal and eloquent in his support of the cigarette tax. Bernie Horn and Len Lucchi, who were working on Muse's campaign, wanted to attack Lawlah for refusing to sign, DeMarco says, but he asked them to hold off until the deadline. He privately urged Lawlah to sign the pledge "so that her opponent could not use her refusal as ammunition, attacking her for taking the side of Big Tobacco against Maryland's children." Lawlah signed just ahead of the deadline and won her race by a hairsbreadth. (In 2005, Lawlah became the lead Senate sponsor for DeMarco's Fair Share Health Care law. In 2006, Lawlah retired from the Senate and Muse took over her Senate seat and became a strong supporter of DeMarco's health-care expansion initiatives.)

On September 4, 1998, the *Baltimore Sun* gave front-page billing to the final pre-election pledge signings: "Anti-Smoking Group Recruits Legislators; 182 Candidates Pledge to Back Cigarette Tax Increase, Coalition Says." The 182 signers included 74 incumbents—"52 house delegates and 22 state senators. Passing the bill would require the votes of 71 delegates and 24 senators." Importantly, the article, by Scott Shane, noted that the signers included the Democratic Senate majority leader, Clarence Blount, and the Republican Senate minority leader, Marty Madden, as well as the House majority leader, John Adams Hurson, and the House Ways and Means Committee chair, Sheila Hixson. It was no surprise that Senate President Mike Miller did not sign, nor did House Speaker Casper Taylor. As the *Sun* story also made clear, DeMarco had not quite corralled the chair "of the other crucial committee for tax legislation," Barbara Hoffman of the Budget and Taxation Committee, who said: "I really don't ever sign pledges, and I think this bill needs a lot of work. But I'm in favor of the tax."

"When this article got published," DeMarco recalls, "I thought we had won. After that, it was just a matter of how much the tax was going to be. We distributed lists of everyone who signed on; everybody sent them everywhere. We're just educating people about who supports the tax and who doesn't. It became an issue all around the state."

5

Politics without Partisanship

As the November general elections approached, DeMarco's challenge was to inflict electoral damage on those candidates who refused to sign the pledge and enhance the electoral chances of those who did. This was no mean task, as MCI was constrained by both its nonprofit tax-exempt status and its nonpartisan credibility, and most of the candidates who did not sign the pledge turned out to be Republicans (although a good number of Republicans did sign it and some Democrats did not). DeMarco had to devise indirect or alternative means for delivering what needed to be, in effect, a partisan message: Do not vote for this candidate; vote for this one.

What made this possible without violating the campaign's restriction on partisan activity was that many candidates, primarily Democrats who signed the pledge, made MCI a campaign issue on their own. Tod Sher, a Democrat, was challenging an incumbent Republican delegate, Patricia Faulkner, a moderate on many issues but who rigidly opposed tobacco tax increases. With advice from Horn and Lucchi, Sher devised a campaign ad picturing a troubled teenage girl smoking a cigarette against a dark background, with the headline, "Don't let her life go up in smoke." Underneath her picture stretched an open cigarette pack on its side, with the (fictitious) label on the box, "WARNING: The Tobacco Industry Is Not Your Friend." And at the bottom: "Neither Is Delegate Faulkner."

No Maryland race was more important to the MCI campaign that year than the governor's—and it was intense and close. "If Ellen Sauerbrey had won," DeMarco says, "there would have been no chance for a tobacco tax increase." So without endorsing Governor Glendening, MCI had to do all it could to highlight Sauerbrey's position on the tobacco tax. One artful tactic was rewarded with this headline in the October 1 *Columbia Flier*: "'Buttman' Shadows Sauerbrey." Buttman, it turned out, was Carole Fisher, "a 63 year old cancer survivor and Democratic activist, already well known as chairwoman of the Howard County Democratic Party." Beside the headline a photo shows Fisher in a cigarette costume, holding a large heart that reads, "Big Tobacco Loves Ellen."

Readers learn that Buttman has appeared at every Sauerbrey rally, asking to meet the candidate. This time, she was waiting in the hotel lobby of a rally, eager only to urge the candidate to sign the pledge: "I'm being her conscience," she told the *Flier*'s reporter. The article recounts that one of Sauerbrey's aides turned Buttman's sign over "so that the words were covered." Then "Vincent DeMarco, Fisher's friend and a major player in the push to make Maryland's cigarette tax the highest in the nation, turned the sign over again."

At this stage of the campaign, the most trusted voices once again were the faith leaders. As a result of Bishop Miles's forceful advocacy, the Interdenominational Ministerial Alliance sponsored a sixty-second radio commercial so controversial that MCI lost some members when it aired, and some people, DeMarco acknowledges, "really chafed" at it but "bit their lips." Strategic Campaign Initiatives, a local consulting firm run by Bernie Horn, Len Lucchi, and Len's wife, Brenda Beitzell, created the radio spot and an accompanying brochure. The commercial's simplicity was elegant, its rhetoric biting, its sound effects devastating. It never mentioned Governor Parris Glendening.

[A voice that could have come from the heavens speaks:]
A message from the Interdenominational Ministerial Alliance.

Guns. *[SFX: Bang]*
Tobacco. *[SFX: Cough]*
Gambling. *[SFX: Ka-ching]*

The rich special interest groups have a candidate who does whatever they want.

Guns. *[SFX: Bang]*
Tobacco. *[SFX: Cough]*
Gambling. *[SFX: Ka-ching]*

It's Ellen Sauerbrey.

The gun lobby. *[SFX: Bang]* They wanted Sauerbrey to vote against every reasonable gun law, including restrictions on semiautomatic assault weapons. And she did.

The big tobacco companies. *[SFX: Cough]* They want Sauerbrey to oppose effective measures to curb teen smoking, such as the Maryland Children's Initiative. And she does.

And the casino gambling interests. *[SFX: Ka-ching]* They want Sauerbrey to stand aside while they fill our state with ten thousand slot machines. And she would.

The rich special interests may control Sauerbrey, but they don't control you. So vote on Tuesday, November 3rd.

[SFX: Bang] [SFX: Cough] [SFX: Ka-ching]

Because Maryland is our state, not theirs.

Grass Roots or Astroturf?

The tobacco lobby, for once, was caught off guard by the media campaign, unused to public interest advocates engaging so aggressively in the political process. Nor would they anticipate the quick reaction time of the MCI team and its close working relationships with key media channels.

Bruce Bereano and his cohorts sorely needed grassroots mobilization to bolster their weakened influence in Annapolis. Two days before the elections, reinforcements arrived in the form of the National Smokers Alliance, which claimed 180,000 irate Maryland smokers as members under the banner "No-strings-attached independence." In a mass mailing designed to infuriate and motivate Maryland smokers to vote against the pledge signers, the alliance warned: "The anti-smokers have come up with yet another way to take our hard-earned money and spend it on more ways to restrict our personal freedom."

The DeMarco team was one step ahead. Glenn Schneider had provided *Baltimore Sun* reporter Scott Shane with copies of once-secret tobacco industry documents exposed through the state attorneys general's litigation against the tobacco companies. When the National Smokers Alliance announced its "grassroots" uprising, two days before the election on November 1, 1998, Shane pounced, under the headline: "Cigarette tax in Md. draws critics to state; Smokers' rights group urging voters to reject backers of higher tax; Links to tobacco industry; Organization asserts it's independent, but documents disagree." Noting that various documents detail the alliance's creation and bankrolling by Philip Morris and a public relations firm, he laid out some facts from the tobacco industry's records: "One 1994 document discloses, in their own words, that the alliance would 'introduce new arguments to confuse the issues and get voters angry.' Another warns that smokers' rights campaigns should be handled by 'Burson-Marsteller [public relations] professionals' and not left to 'locals.'"

Shane disclosed that grassroots members' dues provide less than 1 percent of the alliance's budget. MCI's shocked and on-message response: "'It is reprehensible that a Virginia-based front group for the tobacco industry would try to prevent Marylanders from protecting our children,' says Vincent DeMarco, executive director of the Maryland Children's Initiative, which says the tax would reduce teen smoking." Of the anticipated 180,000 irate Maryland smokers, nineteen Smokers Alliance members called the *Sun* to protest the tax increase. *Sun* reporters were not impressed.

Winning

On Election Day, November 3, sixty-six delegates were elected who had signed the pledge. It would take just five more to reach a majority of the 141 House members. Twenty-three senators were elected who had signed the pledge, just one short of a majority of the Senate's forty-seven members. All four Democratic challengers in Montgomery County who zeroed in on their incumbent Republican opponents' failure to sign the pledge won (including Tod Sher, who had defeated Faulkner, the delegate who was "not your friend"), and each of their votes would be critical in the upcoming 1999 House of Delegates session. Governor Glendening was reelected. He told the *Baltimore Sun*, "I ran on the tobacco tax to protect our children and won big." He would not forget how he won, and he would not forget his pledge.

In the elections, MCI had outflanked a tobacco lobby that, in DeMarco's view, "didn't get it. They weren't paying attention to what we were doing. They weren't lobbying people not to sign." That was because, Bernie Horn observed, "the tobacco industry and other big bad guys hire expensive lobbyists. They don't do grass roots. In their world, you take legislators out to lunch, you wine them and dine them, and that's how you pass legislation. They didn't take this seriously."

Grassroots organizing was certainly not the way Bruce Bereano was used to working (though he did tell me with pride how he organized the tattoo and body-piercing industry in a grassroots coalition to prevent excessive regulation). It was lobbying that Bereano had mastered, with rules learned from many years in Annapolis: "In lobbying, relationships are everything: Are you deferential? Do you know your place?" He faults DeMarco. "There were a number of times when Vinny let his feet get off the ground. He didn't realize he wasn't a senator, wasn't a delegate. He thought he was running the place. It's the legislators' game. We're playing in it, participating, but you've got to know your limitations."

Bereano had failed to recognize that DeMarco's campaign strategies had undermined the effect of even the most skillful traditional lobbyists. Eric Gally, the American Cancer Society lobbyist, reports: "I would get flagged down in the hallways of Annapolis by legislators who said, 'Tell DeMarco to stop getting so many people to call. The phone's ringing off the hook.'" Gally heard stories of legislators getting "four hundred, five hundred, six hundred e-mails and phone calls. These are real people—real people who live in the districts of the legislators they are calling." Bereano is right about one thing, though: DeMarco does not know his limitations.

As the 1999 general session of the Maryland legislature approached, the DeMarco team had reached what appeared to be the peak of their power and prospects for favorable action on the excise tax increase that session. They had the gratitude, vowed support, and political strength of newly elected Governor Glendening. They had 367 member organizations—battle tested in the trenches of the 1998 legislative session and the electoral campaigns at getting the attention of their members' legislators—poised to redeem the pledge those members had made.

Bereano was hardly neutralized, however, and the DeMarco team now had the tobacco companies' attention. Bereano could count on full access to the deep-pocket propaganda and media resources of Philip Morris and its corporate and libertarian think-tank allies, especially in light of a warning in the stockholders' report issued on November 16, 1998: "In the opinion of PM Inc and PMI, past increases in excise and similar taxes have had an adverse impact on the sale of cigarettes. Any future increases, the extent of which cannot be predicted, could result in volume declines for the cigarette industry."

Bereano could call on a team of at least twelve tobacco and allied lobbyists. Though DeMarco's election strategy had caught them napping, they still had many friends in the legislature, not least Senate President Mike Miller; a Democrat, Miller was a critical ally of Governor Glendening on most of the governor's other priorities. The pro-tobacco lobbyists also carried a toolkit newly refurbished with troubling arguments against the tax increase—arguments the industry had honed in beating back President Clinton's effort to raise the federal cigarette tax in 1998. Among these were scientific-sounding declarations about higher cigarette taxes as an incitement to black markets, as indefensible economically, and as ineffectual at reducing cigarette use by kids. Worse, a powerful new tool dropped into the tobacco lobby's hands: an anticipated $1 billion surplus in 1999 state revenues without any tax increases, a windfall fattened by the Maryland attorney general's $4.2 billion share of the

October national settlement of the state attorneys general tobacco company class-action lawsuits.

On November 12, 1998, the *Washington Post* editorial writers fretted that the windfall "could cause problems," not just among anti-tax Republican lawmakers and tobacco farmers. As the *Post* reported, Senate President Miller—again—expressed disdain for any new taxes: "As long as Maryland is a tobacco-growing state, I don't think that we should be the ones that try to tax it out of existence.... As long as we're going to rack up a surplus, there's little sentiment for any tax increase, no matter how onerous the product."

Most legislators who had signed the pledge would not be swayed. The DeMarco team's concern focused on the few who, already eager to turn their backs on the pledge so they could satisfy debts to Bereano and other lobbyists or escape the wrath of Senate President Miller, would now have excuses to do so, as would the uncommitted legislators. Bereano needed only a handful of votes in either house to doom the tax increase.

Stage 5. Pressure for Action

With the January 1999 legislative session in their sights, the DeMarco team launched a postelection campaign that included a media blitz on two fronts: responding aggressively to the tobacco industry's arguments, and holding the pledge signers to their word. The MCI staff prepared what they labeled a call-and-response songbook of compelling rebuttals to each of the industry lobbyists' claims, three to four paragraphs backed by scientific authority. Every MCI spokesperson and advocate would repeat them in every meeting they had with editorial writers and journalists, and in every discussion with legislators.

DeMarco, especially, but also Schneider and other key MCI advocates, could now approach the editorial writers and journalists to whom they had consistently supplied reliable data, good stories, and fuel for appropriate outrage. DeMarco, for instance, again spent considerable time talking with the key editorial writers at the *Baltimore Sun* and the *Washington Post*, both of whom he had worked closely with during the gun control campaign. The results flowed steadily throughout the run-up to the three-month legislative session, which would start serious work by late February.

First came the broadsides from the leading newspapers. On November 14, a *Washington Post* editorial called for the tax increase, claiming that "timing, popular support and legislative momentum are right for enactment of a substantial increase next year in Maryland's cigarette tax." The editorial countered all the arguments—the industry's and Senate President Mike Miller's—and in a final nudge reminded Maryland's top executive of his promise: "Gov. Glendening pledged before his reelection to make enactment a priority—and he should be held to his word."

Swallowing Hard

Barbara Hoffman, chair of the Senate Budget and Taxation Committee, while still a supporter of a higher tax, continued to oppose any bill that wrested power from the committee's hands by dictating the allocation of tax proceeds. Moreover, she thought that distribution of the proceeds favored children's programs too heavily when other priority state needs lacked funding.

DeMarco knew the bill needed Hoffman's support if it was to emerge from her committee, and there was only one way to bring her on board before the 1999 session began: revisit the agreement through which each lead organization in MCI had been guaranteed funding from the tax proceeds for its own priority. DeMarco met separately with each organization's leaders. The Teachers Association, though hardly happy, understood the need for this compromise—and its leaders knew that if the tax increase did pass, it would at least mean more funds in the state budget, which would increase the chances for the association's funding priorities. DeMarco was relieved: "They were still with us." So were the others, except one: Advocates for Children and Youth.

Even if all the coalition's members had agreed, DeMarco knew, changing the bill would give wavering legislators yet another out. The pledge signers had agreed not only to support the $1.50 tax, but also to fund these specific programs, DeMarco said. With that provision changed, he imagined Bereano whispering in legislative ears, "You signed that pledge, but the tax isn't going to fund these programs, so your pledge doesn't really count anymore." Just as he anticipated, some legislators began telling the coalition they no longer felt bound.

A Governor Newly Empowered

Governor Glendening, who along with the Smoke Free Maryland Coalition had been stonewalled during the 1997 session in his quest for a tobacco tax increase, was now a transformed chief executive—far more confident than the Governor Glendening who had squeaked by in the 1994 election, and far more politically surefooted than the Governor Glendening of 1997. His public announcement that the tobacco tax had won him the election came before news of the attorneys general settlement, which he could have claimed raised from tobacco companies far more than the money that the tax would yield, releasing him from his debt to the campaign. "But," said DeMarco, "we reached out to him and said we still need this. He joined us in a press conference, wore one of our stickers, and said, 'Yes, we have this settlement money, but we still need the tobacco tax.'"

The governor would be true to his pledge and his personal commitment to the tax increase, but he did convince DeMarco and his allies that a $1.00 increase, not the initial campaign goal of $1.50, was the best achievable. This was neither a disappointment nor a surprise to DeMarco, who had set the $1.50 goal knowing in his political bones that it would need to be compromised as the campaign progressed. Glendening's rationale was that the recently agreed-to nationwide tobacco settlement had led to a major tobacco price increase, so the campaign could achieve its goal—reducing teen smoking—with just a $1.00 increase. DeMarco points out that it was also "good politics for the governor to show he could successfully negotiate with us before he made his case to the general assembly."

On January 15, just as the assembly session got under way, Glendening presented his proposed state budget, a stick-and-carrot document aimed at any legislator who resisted his $1.00-a-pack tax increase over two years. The budget contained a political mousetrap for legislators looking for a way to avoid voting for the tax: Glendening simply balanced his budget by including the anticipated revenue from the proposed increase. This served notice on the legislators that if they failed to enact the increase, he might be forced to eliminate spending projects—which could coincidentally be projects in districts whose legislators had voted against the tax increase. Even DeMarco's sometime tormentor Senator Barbara Hoffman was finally pleased, she told the *Washington Post's* Daniel LeDuc: "It's an extremely cleverly done budget. All the priorities are right. It does create a constituency for a cigarette tax." To critics of this tobacco tax budget trap, the *Sun* quoted Glendening: "The voters endorsed it in last fall's election."

Turning the Media Volume to Deafening

In January, MCI's media advocacy efforts shifted into high gear again, in sync with a statewide mobilization of its 367 organizations—this time sharply focused on holding legislators to their pledges and pressuring the remaining fence-sitters. Out of a series of press conferences and other events that targeted discrete audiences, perhaps no single story better illustrates the range of messengers and messages than one that appeared on January 9, 1999, in rural, remote Cumberland, Maryland.

Headlined "Group Believes Higher Taxes Way to Curb Smoking," the *Cumberland Times-News* story was prompted by an MCI press conference timed to coincide with the opening of the state legislative session the next week. The news peg was the kickoff of the MCI campaign in Cumberland. The piece opened by identifying the tax initiative as promoted by a "children's advocacy group"—not an anti-smoking group—"working to gather support for an initiative aimed at curbing teen smoking by boosting the Maryland state tax on cigarettes by $1.50 a pack."

The reporter noted that though the event had attracted only a modest audience of twenty, among them were "a large handful of elected officials, including Maryland House Speaker Casper Taylor." He mentioned the spokespeople, all of whom reflected the campaign's focus on children—ministers and teachers. John Riley, president of the Allegany County Teachers Association, whose father died of cancer, called the tax effort "a public health issue." Speaking for the teachers, he said, "As educators, we really felt that we had to be out front." Rev. Jim McMahan, a former smoker, saw young people smoking at Allegany College and said he hoped the initiative would "discourage folks from even considering it."

MCI staff, who were responsible for getting the right people to the press conference, had as usual worked hard to make the event newsworthy, on message, and spontaneous. DeMarco pointed out that they had "found key local representatives of our key statewide groups, the United Methodists and the teachers. The statewide groups helped us find the local people—one more reason that I like to focus on building coalitions of groups, not individuals." He had personally "spent a lot of time cultivating people in the Cumberland area because House Speaker Cas Taylor was from there."

Over the next few weeks, similar launches and similar stories popped up in local papers, as DeMarco had planned, from one end of the state to the other. The DeMarco team's drive lost no fervor as it seamlessly morphed into the governor's campaign for a $1.00 tax increase. A sampling of headlines, spokespeople, and quotations illustrates the relentless pursuit of innovative hooks that the campaign created to gain repeated media attention for what was essentially the same story:

> January 13, the Annapolis *Capital*: "Coalition Urges Tobacco Tax Hike." The hook: The son of a smoking-addicted World War II veteran joins the MCI coalition. Spokesman: DeMarco. "This is the right thing to do from a moral and policy standpoint . . . and from a political standpoint."
>
> January 13, *Baltimore Sun*: "Smoker Owens Backs $1 Cigarette Boost." The hook: A tobacco-addicted tobacco farmer and county executive supports the tax increase. Spokeswoman: county executive Janet Owens. "Anti-smoking advocates found an unusual spokeswoman yesterday to lobby for a proposed increase in the cigarette tax, a tobacco farm owner who is addicted to tobacco use . . . the Anne Arundel County Executive, whose family has raised tobacco for generations in Bristol and who says she and her 18-year-old son smoke." Spokesman: DeMarco. "This is a

horrible addiction, and smokers like the county executive know more than anybody else how difficult it is to stop. We do not consider the tobacco farmers in any way our enemy. They are stuck in the middle like everyone else. We applaud Janet Owens for sticking up for what's right."

January 26, *Baltimore Sun*: "Legislators, Teens, Seek Increase in Cigarette Tax." The hook: Teenagers affected by tobacco use favor the tax increase. Spokespeople: The teenagers themselves. "Kicking off a grass-roots campaign for a $1-a-pack increase in the state cigarette tax, Howard County activists employed a new weapon yesterday in their battle against the tobacco industry: children." Spokesman: Joel Lapin, whose wife had died the previous September of lung cancer at the age of forty-nine. "Please, for those that love you and for those you love, do two things. Continue your pledge not to smoke and do the right thing." Spokesman: DeMarco. "They used to say that it was a politically difficult thing to vote against tobacco. Legislators, it's a politically difficult thing to vote against the citizens."

January 26, *Washington Post*: "County Leaders Fired Up about Tobacco Tax Plan." The hook: Influential county leaders endorse what had now become "Glendening's proposed tax increase." Spokesman: DeMarco. "We think legislators pay attention to local officials, especially county leaders."

January 30, op-ed, *Baltimore Afro-American*: "Support Tobacco Tax; Say 'No' to Lobbyists." The hook: Smoking hurts the poor more than a tax increase would. ("The tobacco industry argues that a higher tax will hurt poor people, but we argue that smoking hurts poor people much more.") Spokesman: Bishop Douglas Miles. "When one tobacco executive was asked how young they should go after potential smokers, his answer was, 'If they've got lips, we want them.'"

A One-Two Punch: A Poll and a Rally

As the session approached, Cancer Society lobbyist Eric Gally had felt daunted "because it was a giant mountain to climb and tax increases rarely passed. But by the time the session started, we had probably done 80 percent of our work." That January, he found a welcome contrast in atmosphere from earlier efforts to increase tobacco taxes. "It was a great thing to get to Annapolis as a lobbyist and find legislators coming up to you and feeling that they had to say something about the tax. The buzz in Annapolis was the tobacco tax. Soon the discussion became how much of a tax, not whether."

The momentum caught up even DeMarco's family. As the legislative session progressed, DeMarco took his son Tony's Cub Scout pack to Annapolis to meet with their delegate, Talmadge Branch. Branch had never signed the pledge. "After a few softball questions from parents," DeMarco reports, "Tony asked him, 'Where do you stand on the tobacco tax issue?' in front of a few dozen voting parents from his district. Taken aback, Delegate Branch said, 'Well, I guess I am for it.'"

On February 9, MCI released yet another poll, again by a joint team of Democratic and Republican pollsters. This poll dealt with voters' reactions to the huge payments to the state from the attorneys general settlement. The pollsters' conclusion, reported by the *Baltimore Sun* and other papers: "Hearing about the Maryland settlement does not inhibit support for higher taxes to help control teen smoking. If anything, the tobacco settlement encourages public support for tobacco control measures of all types including taxation.... By a two-to-one margin, Maryland voters favor a $1.00 per pack increase in the cigarette tax as part of an effort to reduce teen smoking." Later, the campaign would break the poll results down and along with supporters from each county hold press conferences in county seats. There they would announce the backing of the county's voters for the tax, providing fresh news for county and regional papers—and hard-to-ignore data for local legislators now in Annapolis.

Next, the campaign scheduled a rally for February 16 that made news even before it took place. The February 12 issue of the *Baltimore Sun* in its "Assembly Digest" carried the headline "Clergy Pledges to Unite for Cigarette Tax." The story was that "Maryland religious leaders pledged yesterday to mobilize their congregations to attend an Annapolis rally Monday in support of a proposed $1-a-pack cigarette tax increase." The same day, the *Baltimore Times* reported, under the headline "Anti-Teen Smoking Tax Favored": "On February 4, dozens of pastors from around Baltimore joined the Interdenominational Ministerial Alliance and the Maryland Children's Initiative in welcoming Lt. Governor Kathleen Kennedy Townsend at the Great Blacks in Wax Museum." On that highly symbolic site, "they called upon the Maryland General Assembly to pass a $1.00 per pack increase in the state's cigarette tax to reduce teen smoking. They also called on citizens to join them in a rally in front of the State House in Annapolis on February 16 at 5:30 p.m."

The rally ratcheted up the pressure on the legislature by manifesting in its breadth and passion the intensity of support for the tax increase. It was a boisterous affair, especially since Selywn Ray from MCI's key partner group the Safe and Sound Campaign had prepared a one-page sheet tailored to a range of expressive modes, "Rally Chants, Rap, and Song." On February 16, the *Capital Gazette* printed a long front-page story with four photographs, its headline quoting one of the chants: "Pass the Bill. Tobacco Can Kill; Marchers Support $1 Cigarette Tax." The lead: "Hundreds of supporters of a measure that would hike Maryland's cigarette tax by $1 a pack swarmed into Annapolis last night, bringing traffic to a standstill ... as proponents marched on the State House, ... students, teachers, church groups and medical professionals." MCI had lit the signal fires. It was time for the legislature to act.

Rebellion in the Ranks

DeMarco had thus far succeeded in keeping the MCI coalition intact and energized despite the loss of guaranteed funding for each member's priority programs. But Advocates for Children and Youth, the only one of the original lead organizations that refused to go along with dropping the bill's mandatory allocation of the tax proceeds, persisted in offering its own amendment to the tax bill. This posed a double threat: to the unity of the coalition and to the still precarious legislative support for the bill.

DeMarco swallows many frustrations and disappointments, and his anger rarely surfaces. Yet with the defection of Advocates for Children and Youth, he says, he "almost went through the roof."

> They had done nothing but cause me grief. Then they were preparing to come to the legislative hearings to testify in favor of the bill—with an amendment: to devote one-third of the tobacco tax to their programs. I said, "Have you talked with anybody about this? Have you talked to the governor's office?" No, they hadn't talked to the governor's office about it. I was livid. "What? You can't do that." Then they started getting tricky. They said they had talked to Eric Gally. He said no, they had talked to him about getting a third of the settlement funds, and he had told them no.
>
> I called them up and said, "If I hear this on the floor of the House; if I hear a delegate referring to this document ..." I told them to just stay out of it. They wanted this money from the tobacco tax, but they weren't willing to work to get the tobacco tax passed. I said, "If you kill the bill, you're not going to get any money anyway."

In the end, Advocates for Children and Youth dropped its proposed amendment. Over time, DeMarco let go of his anger, and the organization would again become what he would call a "stalwart" partner in his future tobacco tax increase and health-care expansion campaigns.

The initiative could now count on close to a majority in the House—those who had signed the pledge—as well as strong leadership from the House Ways and Means Committee chair and a clear majority vote from committee members. Yet passage on the House floor remained in doubt on two counts: the opposition of the House speaker, Casper Taylor, and the continued fierce lobbying by Bereano's team and countless other back-scratching and sympathetic business and labor lobbyists. Nonetheless, on March 26, 1999, the $1.00-per-pack increase passed the 141-member House by four votes.

Four Factors

This signal victory, though only in one house of the legislature, marks a good place to pause to weigh the four factors most critical to the 1999 House vote. The first was the two years spent organizing the largest coalition of engaged citizen groups on record in the state, making the election pledge campaign so formidable. Only one delegate who had signed the pledge voted against the increase; the rest formed the critical base that passed the bill.

The second factor, and the essential complement to the organizing, was the incessant drumbeat of the campaign's media advocacy—for almost two years an interweaving of earned news stories, early seeded and nurtured editorial support, letters to the editor, and planted op-ed articles—which came to a crescendo on the eve of the 1999 legislative session. On the very morning of the House vote, the *Baltimore Sun* ran an op-ed piece by the head of the Maryland Center for Poverty Solutions, Robert Hess, who argued persuasively that increasing tobacco taxes helped lower-income people by saving their lives. Glenn Schneider had drafted the piece and had asked Hess to submit it, knowing that the tax's effect on the poor was a key argument against it. One of the bill's primary backers, Delegate Salima Marriott of Baltimore City, read that op-ed aloud on the floor during the vote.

The third critical factor was the unrelenting lobbying by MCI partners up to the moment of the vote. On April 1, 1999, the *Sun*'s Fraser Smith captured its unique nature:

> A legion of no-name advocates has descended on the Assembly: Knots of clergymen weighed down with brilliant pink or yellow handouts have been standing in doorways looking for legislators throughout the session. They have been joined by students, survivors of smoking's victims, county executives and lobbyists for an array of social issues.
>
> Once the pushovers of the tobacco wars—taunted as health police by some of the tobacco lobbyists—the coalition includes 360 community groups, 7,000 Maryland physicians, national health organizations willing to spend big dollars, 600 high schools and middle schools, and two beauty queens.

The fourth factor was the passion and political skill of Governor Parris Glendening and the equally committed one-on-one lobbying of Lieutenant Governor Kathleen Kennedy Townsend. Grudging respect for the governor's efforts came from an unlikely source. Tobacco Institute lobbyist Bill Pitcher, an old friend of DeMarco's from Young Democrats days, told the *Baltimore Sun*: "There's nothing we can offer to match what the governor can give. The way the governor has intertwined the tax revenue with every legislator's project, it looks like he's giving away that money two or three times."

Glendening "called individual legislators," marvels longtime lobbyist Eric Gally. "Called them in one by one and said, 'If you want this road?' 'If you want this bridge?' 'If you want this elementary school?' 'If you want'—whatever it is they wanted—'you will vote for this bill.' And he told people who had pet bills that had already passed, 'If you don't want me to veto your bill, you'll vote for this bill.' He used all the extraordinary powers the Maryland constitution grants him to drag us across the finish line." But even this factor was not independent of the MCI campaign, for what sealed Glendening's passionate commitment was the campaign's decisive influence on his reelection, as it turned the spotlight on challenger Ellen Sauerbrey's anti-tobacco tax and other seamy special interest vulnerability.

6

Victory and Accountability

Within ten days of the House vote, articles in the *Baltimore Sun* and the *Washington Post* documented MCI's unprecedented visibility and power. Three veteran political analysts who had closely followed the initiative reflected on the changed political environment—to DeMarco's delight (and not without his influence). On April 1, 1999, the *Sun*'s C. Fraser Smith, his early skepticism abating, wrote a column headlined "Tobacco's Lobby Wilting as Grass Roots Reach Deep; In Annapolis, Power Shifts toward $1 Boost in Cigarette Tax." On April 6, the *Washington Post* ran a story and analysis by Saundra Torry and Daniel LeDuc: "Tobacco Battle Too Close to Call; Smoking Foes Show Muscle in Assembly Fight over Tax Hike."

The journalists could not resist the obvious metaphor. The *Sun*'s Smith: "After years of supremacy in the General Assembly, lobbyists for the Goliath of Big Tobacco could be felled this year by the David of grass-roots opposition." The *Washington Post*'s Torry and LeDuc: "No longer a midget flinging itself against Big Tobacco, the anti-smoking movement has grown increasingly sophisticated in Maryland, where it has built a broad network of supporters, flexed its election-year muscles and spent $300,000 on a television and radio campaign in recent weeks."

Still, the vote in the House had been close, and some of the pledge makers shaky. The Senate, under the iron hand of Mike Miller, had all along posed the main obstacle.

The Senate

In the Senate Budget and Taxation Committee, the Glendening political juggernaut ran head-on into Mike Miller. The collision prompted a scathing April 7 editorial in the *Post* that called upon legislators to keep focused on "the difference between a serious move to discourage smoking and a cave-in to tobacco interests seeking a pointlessly weak increase or no bill at all" and suggested that "members of the committee who give serious thought" to the "costly damages of smoking" ought to "see the proposal into law."

During hearings on the tax increase, committee chair Barbara Hoffman indulged in one light moment that signaled a change of atmosphere in the Senate, where lobbyist Bruce Bereano had long held power. Now won over by DeMarco's concession not to mandate the allocation of the tax proceeds, "she was now very much on our side," DeMarco says. "Proponents present their case first, and she gave us lots of time." Bereano, scheduled to be the first witness for the opposition, had to get back to the halfway house where he had been confined following his criminal conviction for political funding abuses. With time running out, he had just scurried out of the hearing room as Hoffman began calling the opposition witnesses. "When she called up Bruce Bereano," says DeMarco, "somebody else came up to testify. 'Where is Mr. Bereano?' she asked, feigning innocence. The witness answered sheepishly, 'He had a previous engagement.' And everybody knew where, and the room burst into howls of laughter."

Yet Hoffman had to struggle mightily to come up with a seven-vote majority to get a tax increase—any tax increase—out of her committee. The campaign was on the brink of failure, just as in 1997. As the April 8 vote of the committee loomed, DeMarco ally Chris Van Hollen and Hoffman had nailed down only six votes. The holdout was Senator Gloria Lawlah of Prince George's County, a profile in ambivalence.

Lawlah "recently received a stack of preprinted cards from tax opponents, but those aren't on her mind as decision time nears," reported *Washington Post* writers Torry and LeDuc in their April 6 story. The governor, pressing her for support, she said, had asked her, "'what are you really interested in?' I said, 'Governor, I've always been interested in Rosecroft,'" a raceway that had long been an economic mainstay of Lawlah's impoverished district. The article went on: "Last week, the governor announced plans to provide $10 million to bolster purses for the harness track at Rosecroft and at Maryland's thoroughbred tracks." But Lawlah still held out, feeling "tugged in the opposite direction. Sitting in the empty Senate chamber Friday, she looked toward the chair from which Senate President Miller presides" and told the reporters, "'Mike Miller is responsible for me being in leadership. I want to see what Mike wants.' . . . 'He holds the key.'"

Lawlah paid little attention to the editorials from the *Sun* or the *Post* or others from outside her district, but she was plainly rattled by the attention her pledge received from the local papers. The April 7 *Prince George's Journal* focused on her backing away from the pledge under a front-page headline, "Senator Now Wavering on Tobacco Tax," and highlighted her exceedingly lame quote: "I signed the pledge, but I also have the right to change my mind." It got worse for the senator in the body of the story. "Lawlah refused to say whether she is supporting the tobacco tax or not. In earlier interviews, Lawlah suggested that DeMarco and his group were attempting to hold her to her earlier pledge," the *Journal* reported. "'I pledged to vote the $1 tax, but I certainly hope they are not trying to hold that over me,' Lawlah said Friday. 'What are they going to do, throw me in jail?' Lawlah said that after 'January 1, reality sets in and you have to look around.'"

DeMarco, quoted in the same article, chose the carrot rather than the stick: "We hope she will support the tobacco tax because it will save the lives of children in Maryland. We know Senator Lawlah cares about the lives of children." The paper followed up this piece a few days later with a scalding op-ed column titled, "When Is a Promise Not a Promise?" by a former member of the Maryland House. The author concluded: "So Gloria, what is a pledge? It is defined as 'a solemn promise or agreement to do or refrain from doing something.' Certainly you have the right to change your mind. And your constituents should be able to change their minds, too. But the Maryland Constitution doesn't contain a recall provision."

Just before the committee vote, the governor published his supplemental budget. Among money earmarked for various projects funded by a cigarette tax increase was the $10 million Lawlah had coveted for Rosecroft racetrack. Still pulling her loyalties in the other direction was Senate President Miller, who parked himself in the room during the Budget and Taxation Committee vote. Neither the full force of the governor's largess nor the voices of Lawlah's constituents could neutralize the force of Miller's power. Hoffman could get only five members of her committee to vote for the one-dollar increase. Lawlah was not among them. But Hoffman did get a majority of seven votes, including Lawlah's, for a thirty-six-cent increase, which the committee sent to the Senate floor. DeMarco and Governor Glendening were stoic. They had almost failed to get any significant increase out of the committee.

Filibuster

Twenty-three of the twenty-four senators whose votes were necessary to pass the bill had signed the pledge, and the governor's budgetary legerdemain had secured the votes of others. When hard-line Republican opponents were threatening to filibuster to prevent the bill from coming to a vote on the

Senate floor, Senate President Mike Miller assured the *Post*'s LeDuc that he "would work to stop any filibuster," apparently resigned to the thirty-six-cent increase. Still, as the assembly session drew to a close, a small group of Republican senators declared that they would go ahead with their plan to stop the tax increase.

Their leader was Senator Robert R. Neall from Anne Arundel County, who, according to the *Baltimore Sun*'s later report, "cracked the whip on the Assembly's strongest filibuster effort in recent years." Their goal was to talk, if necessary, to the last minute of the ninety-day session, midnight on Monday, April 12, at which point it would be too late to vote. The filibuster started Wednesday afternoon, April 7, with Neall and his cadre proposing and discussing amendment after amendment. Despite Miller's pledge, says Glenn Schneider, he allowed the "filibustering senators to go home and sleep until one of our advocates, Senator Paul Pinsky, asked out loud why the Senate president was aiding and abetting a Republican filibuster."

Once again, Governor Glendening went to work. He needed to win over the four tobacco-district Democrats who had been holding out to cut the tax increase to twenty-five cents. In what seemed an endless series of meetings in a room behind the Senate chamber, he finally persuaded the holdouts to supply the missing four votes for a thirty-cent increase.

That further cut infuriated DeMarco's colleagues. "Chris Van Hollen came out during the filibuster and told us that we needed to make a decision," Schneider says. "Should he kill the bill if it's only thirty cents?" This was one time DeMarco let his eagerness to win something worthwhile cloud his judgment. "Vinny was sick when Eric and I asked Chris to push for more," says Schneider. Their feeling was that if they couldn't get "the whole thing," they should "at least try to get a commitment from the assembly to put significant money toward tobacco use prevention and cessation. Without it, we agreed to speak of the end result with little but faint praise."

The Senate passed the bill with the thirty-cent-per-pack increase, 29–18, at 8:30 p.m. on April 10. Schneider credits Chris Van Hollen, who "used his amazing skills to guarantee a complete victory, getting $21 million for the tobacco control programs. Thirty cents and tobacco prevention dollars made us giddy. It was the first time that any state passed a tobacco tax solely for health reasons and not to satisfy a budget deficit." Yet, after two years of relentless, skillful advocacy, with massive outside pressure, and fierce inside advocates, the power of one determined foe in the Senate, President Miller, was sufficient to reduce the campaign's victory by two-thirds.

After the vote, DeMarco's comment to the *Sun* was uncharacteristically subdued: "This package will save some lives."

Stage 6. Accountability

The MCI campaign was ready to shut down, but Vinny DeMarco was not. "The filibuster was a horrible thing," he said, outraged. "All they talked about was the horror of tobacco, but their goal was to kill the bill at the bidding of the tobacco lobby. I kept thinking about Marsha Lapin." Lapin had testified for the tax increase as she was dying of lung cancer. "There would be so many fewer tragedies like Marsha's if this bill passed. It's one thing to vote against it, but to filibuster is a different story."

A *Washington Post* story by Amy Argetsinger about the leader of the filibuster, Senator Neall, fueled DeMarco's anger. The piece appeared the day after the vote, April 11, headlined "Senate GOP's Onetime Star Rises Again in Md. Assembly" and quoting Ray Feldmann, Glendening's press secretary: "'The governor respects Bobby Neall. He played a significant role in all this and it was not unexpected given his experience. He's one of the Republican senators the governor respects.'"

This was too much for DeMarco, who felt "like so many people in Maryland had thought about this issue because of our work. We wanted people to know these senators were using a filibuster against it." He points out that data a few years later showed that "twenty thousand fewer kids smoked. A third would have died horrible deaths. We were absolutely right about what we were doing. And that filibuster came within minutes and seconds of killing the bill, so I thought it was critical that people know."

DeMarco also wanted to make sure that Neall and his colleagues paid a political price for their actions and that in any of his own future campaigns, no legislators would be tempted to follow their example. With MCI Board approval, he turned to Bernie Horn and Len Lucchi. He at first did not want to run the radio ad Horn developed, Bernie says, because "he knew that he was going to get a lot of grief." DeMarco muses that the only time he ever got a call from Senate President Mike Miller was when Miller got wind that he was planning to run the ad. Miller urged him not to use it, and DeMarco told him, "I can't do that—I had a hard enough time convincing people not to include you in the ad."

According to Horn, Lucchi told DeMarco he had to do it. "They've got to be afraid of you. Who the hell are you? You've got to tell them who the hell you are." Horn points out that "it's a whole lot easier for me and Len to say, 'Do this.' Nobody blames us." But they felt that "if Vinny was going to have any weight, he had to show what he could do. We gave him good political advice. And he took it, which was very difficult."

This was the final version of the ad:

Announcer: A message from the Maryland Children's Initiative.
   [SFX: background noise of children on a playground]
Child One: Ahh . . . Billy.
Child Two: I'll take . . . Suzie.
Child One: Joey.
Child Two: Mary.
   [SFX: background noise fades]
Announcer: Choosing sides . . . What if adults choose sides AGAINST kids?
   [SFX: background noise of legislators]
Clerk: Senator Neall.
Voice One: No.
Clerk: Senator Harris.
Voice Two: No.
Clerk: Senator Jacobs.
Voice Three: No.
   [SFX: background noise fades out]
Announcer: It happened in Annapolis.
   A bill to increase the price of cigarettes by 30 cents a pack came to the
   Senate floor. Experts estimated it would save the lives of 8,000 children
   in our state.
   One group stubbornly opposed the bill—the big tobacco companies.
   And when the State Senators chose sides, a small number—including
   Robert Neall, Andrew Harris, and Nancy Jacobs—turned their backs on
   our kids.
   Arm-in-arm with the tobacco lobbyists, they led a desperate filibuster.
   Fortunately, they lost.
   So next time you're asked to choose sides . . .
   [SFX: background noise for legislators]
Clerk: Senator Neall.
Voice One: No.
Clerk: Senator Harris.
Voice Two: No.
Clerk: Senator Jacobs.
Voice Three: No.
   [SFX: background noise fades out]
Announcer: Think about it.

Five of the filibusterers were targeted in separate broadcasts of the ad in
two parts of the state. Naturally, the targets of the ads, and Republicans generally, erupted in outrage. But so did one of DeMarco's closest allies, among the

staunchest supporters of the campaign, the Maryland State Medical Society, or MedChi. "Batting Heads over an Ad," ran a May 11 *Baltimore Sun* headline. "MedChi, the Maryland State Medical Society, disassociated itself from the Maryland Children's Initiative last week," the article reported, and in a letter to DeMarco, MedChi "called the ads 'unwise and counterproductive,'" demanding that their "name be removed from all Maryland Children's Initiative literature."

This followed by one day, the article went on, Senate Minority Leader Martin G. Madden's denouncement of DeMarco as "a partisan mouthpiece for the Democrats" because the ad's targeted senators were all Republicans. "Madden erupted after the *Sun* reported last week that DeMarco was planning an attack on Republican lawmakers over their tobacco tax votes." The piece quoted DeMarco, "a man who could find the bright side of an Internal Revenue Service audit": "'I understood that maybe not every one of our groups would agree with this strategy,' DeMarco said. But he said he and the Children's Initiative board decided the public needed to know who led the filibuster." He then went on the offensive: "I consider the filibuster hardball," he told the *Sun*. "If there had been no filibuster, there would be no ad."

MedChi's recoil from the ad was inevitable: the Medical Society had too many issues constantly before the legislature, and the group would need—and have a good shot at—the votes of these very filibusterers for some of these issues. The physicians could not afford to make them permanent enemies. But DeMarco and MCI had only one issue: getting the tax increase passed. Since MCI would go out of business when that job was done, the only remaining target for the filibusterers' revenge was DeMarco, and he could not conceive of any future campaign in which these five could be allies.

Measuring the Achievement

The effect of the thirty-cent increase and of the 1999 bill's other tobacco control provisions was manifest a little more than a year later. On August 26, 2000, the *Baltimore Sun* reported: "Sharp Drop in Cigarette Sales in State; 16 Percent Decrease in 2000 Was Biggest Decline in 20 Years." The experts disagreed over how to distribute the credit for this decrease among the state excise tax increase, cigarette price rises that resulted from the costs of the litigation settlement, and cross-border smuggling from low-tax Virginia. But most agreed the tax increase had made a difference.

One man had no doubts, as the *Sun* reported: "Vincent DeMarco, who organized the campaign to increase the state cigarette tax, noted that nearly 60 million fewer packs were sold this fiscal year than last." In his comment, Vinny stayed on message. "'That's a tremendous achievement,' he said. 'Clearly, we're saving lives.'"

On October 20, 2001, in an editorial that praised the results of the continuing drop in cigarette sales, the *Sun* commented: "It's difficult to think of a public health measure that could match the contribution of the thirty-cent-per-pack tax increase." In 2002, an election year, the General Assembly passed an additional thirty-four-cent cigarette tax to fund education. There was no filibuster.

Part II

Health Care for More:
The Chameleon Campaign

In his first meeting with the Smoke Free Maryland Board following the 1997 legislative session, DeMarco had presented a remarkably comprehensive plan based on the strategies he had developed during ten years of trial and not much error in six successful gun control campaigns. Despite a bump or two, that was the plan the DeMarco team followed to a successful conclusion in 1999 for the cigarette tax increase. Several factors helped make that campaign achievable: a relatively simple objective with multiple beneficiaries, a black-hat adversary the public had learned to scorn, no major unforeseen calamities, and a potent inside leader in the governor. But how would DeMarco lead a campaign in which none of these factors was present?

For the next ten years, beginning in 1999, DeMarco led what became a series of campaigns in which he confronted multiple barriers. The issue that would engage him was health-care expansion at the state level. In Part I, I followed chronologically the course of the MCI campaign and the full deployment of DeMarco's strategic template. Though DeMarco would continue to apply that template, in Part II I narrow the focus to how he responded to challenges not present in the MCI campaign.

7

An Impossible Dream?

In the spring of 1999, in the midst of the legislative session, Vincent DeMarco had only one goal in mind: get the tobacco tax passed. So focused was he that, he confesses, he "had no idea and no plan for what to do next." But if he was not thinking of his next campaign, that campaign was thinking of him. Not a coalition, this time, but one passionate advocate: Dr. Peter Beilenson, the health commissioner of Baltimore.

At the time, Beilenson says, "I frankly could not believe that we could continue to allow ourselves to be one of three major countries left in the world—Turkey and Mexico being the others—that do not have universal health coverage. Yet we're the wealthiest, most technologically advanced country in the world. It is simply unconscionable. There were seven hundred thousand people in Maryland then who did not have health insurance, and another seven or eight hundred thousand who had such poor health coverage that they couldn't afford primary preventive care."

Informally, Beilenson had begun to convene other health-care advocates who had lobbied in Annapolis, year after year, for even incremental improvements in health-care coverage for Maryland's citizens, with little success. He had also mobilized a team of ten or so public health professionals in his own department to come up with far broader reforms and a more muscular strategy. They were "good-guy granola types" with their hearts in the right place—but not strategists, he acknowledged. At one of their meetings, Carol Beck from the Abell Foundation suggested that they needed a Vinny DeMarco.

Beilenson had worked in harmony with DeMarco on the gun control and tobacco tax campaigns. He also sensed that DeMarco "was about to be successful again and work himself out of a job because the tobacco tax was about to pass." Beilenson read DeMarco as an advocate who "seemed to have a very successful template for social change through the political process" and had twice watched him successfully apply that template, though Beilenson acknowledged that health-care reform was a much more complex issue than either gun control or tobacco. Despite the complexity, DeMarco, who had never advocated professionally for health care, was intrigued by the prospect and agreed to explore partnering with Beilenson to lead a new campaign to achieve health care for all Marylanders.

Not yet forty, Beilenson had been health commissioner for eight years under two strong-minded mayors. Like DeMarco, he is passionate about his causes, but where DeMarco is cautious and disciplined in his public statements, the Harvard-educated Beilenson is sometimes less than diplomatic, though eloquent. Thus *Baltimore Sun* writer Michael Ollove reported in an October 1, 2000, profile of the health commissioner: "It is his experience that only 20 percent of the population is competent in what they do. Recently he has halved that estimate. In his department, he says, bureaucratic ineptitude is as entrenched as disease in the greater community." Ollove describes Beilenson as "tall, stringy, prematurely bald, but with the agility of a collegian."

Beilenson told about a hundred Democratic staff members at a hearing on Capitol Hill, Ollove wrote, "that he expects to do what President Clinton and Hillary Rodham Clinton could not. That he will rally a notoriously cantankerous medical profession. That he will persuade notoriously weak-willed legislators. That he will take on the formidable resources of the insurance companies, and win."

DeMarco was no stranger to strong-minded partners, nor averse to optimism. He told Beilenson that he was ready to proceed, but cautioned that if the public will was not there for fundamental change, it would be folly to press ahead.

The Challenge of Complexity

Almost everyone, even most smokers, opposed smoking by kids; the only complex policy issues in the tobacco tax campaign had been, how high should we raise the tax? and who's going to get the money? Similarly, almost every analyst who seriously looked at U.S. health care—that is, every analyst neither fettered with free-market ideological blinders nor profiting from the present system—agreed with Beilenson's harsh assessment: the system was unconscionable. But health care was not tobacco; there was no consensus on what to do about health care, or on how to achieve health care for all.

The biggest challenge for a campaign would be the deep schism among health-care advocates over the best route to health care for all. A small but passionate constituency was determined to replace the current jerry-built system of health-care financing dominated by private insurers with a single-payer root-and-branch revolution through which one source—the federal government or a subcontracting entity—would pay for everyone's health care using mandatory tax revenues. Other reformers saw the single-payer system as a politically unattainable fantasy and advocated a spectrum of reforms, including incremental expansion of Medicare and Medicaid, but not abrupt replacement of the current system.

If that dissention weren't daunting enough, anyone who tried to achieve comprehensive reform in 1999 would face a series of other formidable political obstacles. Since the Clintons' health-care initiative had collapsed ignominiously earlier in the decade, the political energy for broad health-care reform had languished, even among progressive politicians. Republicans, also in thrall to a conservative free-market ideology that despised government intervention in all but war, were in raucous ascendancy, even in traditionally Democratic Maryland. There, as we have seen, a progressive governor had a hard time being reelected against a defiantly right-wing, corporate-courting opponent.

Private health insurers and others who profited most from the defects in the U.S. health-care system—not nearly so universally reviled as the tobacco merchants of death—could call on an armory of economic and political resources. They had demonstrated in the Clinton battles skillful deployment of those resources and were ever at the ready for combat. Furthermore, the decade had witnessed a wholesale turnover of nonprofit Blue Cross and other health insurance plans to profit-seeking entrepreneurs, who were also politically fortified to defend their investments.

Also armed for battle were the leaders of the business community, small and large, conditioned by decades of libertarian rhetoric from the American Medical Association to rise up at the specter of "socialized medicine." (Business owners were not yet balking at international competition from companies whose employee health benefits were borne by their governments.) Any health-care expansion would cost public money and strain tight state budgets; fundamental reform would push them to the breaking point. No wonder DeMarco expressed caution.

Running the Numbers: Funding and Polling

DeMarco and Beilenson asked Robert Embry of the Abell Foundation for $100,000, more than DeMarco had ever sought before. Half would support a broader, more in-depth poll than DeMarco had ever done, with follow-up research, carried out by a leading—and expensive—national pollster, Robert

Green of Penn, Schoen and Berland Associates. The second $50,000 would mostly pay DeMarco's salary. (Some other funds Beilenson had already raised could pay for recruiting a new team to run the campaign.)

Embry was skeptical. Although he strongly supported universal health care, he asked: "How could this be possible in light of the Clinton failure? This could be money down the tubes." When DeMarco responded that he would be able to build on the base of the gun and tobacco coalitions, Embry took a "leap of faith," says DeMarco. The Abell Board approved the grant.

"And I have to immediately write a check for most of it to the polling firm," says DeMarco, "when I'm not even assured of my salary. I'm thinking, 'Is this a huge mistake?' But I can't emphasize enough: you have to do a poll. People would say, 'What are you going to do if the poll doesn't show support?' And I'd have to say, 'Then we can't go forward with it.'" The poll was designed to answer a series of key questions: Do a strong majority of voters care about universal health care? If so, do they care enough? How would they feel about having their current coverage converted by government action into something different, for instance, into a government-run or mandated program? Which changes would they support energetically, which merely superficially? Which would they barely tolerate, and which resist?

The results in the summer of 1999 showed that the seed investment had paid off. The numbers "surprised me more than any poll I'd done," DeMarco marvels. "It was an overwhelming 80 percent of support for health care for all." For DeMarco, as always, "the most important question was testing the political strength of the issue. This poll showed a substantial shift in voter intent depending on a candidate's support [for] or opposition to health care for all. This showed me the potential of this being a tremendously powerful political issue—a resounding yes, the issue can work." The campaign would go forward.

Yet, given the formidable complexity of the search for a politically viable health policy for the uninsured, DeMarco and Beilenson decided, with input from DeMarco's brain trust, that this campaign would modify DeMarco's template. First, they would stay away from the legislature, not for just one or two years, but for four years, which they would devote to developing the optimal health-care plan and the public education needed to mobilize support for it. Second, they would build a coalition bigger and broader than any of those in earlier campaigns; they would need more money, and new allies.

Beyond polling, organizing, media advocacy, and other now standard elements of the DeMarco template, they would directly seek to uncover stakeholders' and concerned citizens' hopes and fears about potential ways to expand health-care coverage. They would engage authoritative health policy experts to help transform public will into technically workable and politically achievable legislation. They would also engage unimpeachable economic experts to explore and then make the case that universal health-care coverage was economically feasible at the state level.

Listening

One reason DeMarco hesitated to announce at the outset the campaign's commitment to a single-payer system lay imbedded in the poll results: people who had health insurance from private insurers overwhelmingly wanted to hold tight to that insurance. When they expressed a desire to see universal coverage, they were talking about helping others—the poor and uninsured—get health care and about reducing health-care costs for themselves.

DeMarco would not advance a plan that held no hope of gathering broad public support. He and Beilenson agreed to talk to and, more important, to listen to as many concerned people as possible. Through the remainder of 1999, they would continue the conversations with Beilenson's Health Department staff and frustrated health-care reform activists, and broaden their outreach to public health advocates and citizen activists. Glenn Schneider would soon join the effort, and if he hesitated before committing himself to another DeMarco rollercoaster, DeMarco never once considered going forward without Schneider: "When Peter Beilenson asked me to take on the health issue, it was a no-brainer for me to reach out to Glenn to join me in a key role. He became the backbone of our organization, making the computers—our trains— run on time, being our chief policy person on health issues (which he came to know as well as he always knew tobacco issues), overseeing staff and consultants, and otherwise being central to our successes. The board and our coalition partners all loved working with him."

Beilenson, DeMarco, Schneider, Beilenson's Health Department staff members, and a few other key players would continue to meet separately, strategize, plan next steps, tap DeMarco and Beilenson's funding contacts, and debate the merits of competing policy solutions. Among participants in these early meetings, the single-payer solution was by far the favored route to pursue.

Over the next two years, 2000 and 2001, these strategy meetings would gradually broaden to include discrete constituencies that needed to be heeded to ensure that the plan ultimately campaigned for would not only secure the grand goal of health care for all, but also be financially practicable. For DeMarco, the sine qua non would be to assure sufficiently broad political support to give a fighting chance for legislative success within a reasonable time frame. These core constituencies would include:

Stakeholders whose professional lives were entwined with the present
   system, and who would be most affected by change: professional groups
   representing hospitals, doctors, nurses, social workers, labor, and business. Meetings with stakeholders would be designed to tease out each
   group's real hopes and fears—and to gauge the intensity of these feelings.
Advocates for children, mental health, community health centers, substance
   abuse treatment, and alternative medicine.
Government officials who directed and monitored health-care programs,
   who could subvert any plan that made life a headache for them.
Potential leaders and partner organizations for a new coalition, starting with
   many of those who had formed the core of DeMarco's gun control and
   tobacco tax coalitions, particularly the faith community.
Engaged members of the public—citizens who cared enough about the holes
   in the health-care safety net to show up at town meetings around the
   state, who would be encouraged to share their concerns regarding their
   experiences with the current health-care delivery system, along with
   their questions about and suggestions for reform under a new system.
   They, too, would have to be convinced that the solution the initiative
   offered would address their concerns without creating new ones.

Bringing in the Experts

Simultaneously, DeMarco and Beilenson needed to engage a team of
credentialed experts, again unlike the tobacco campaign, where expert scientific opinion (independent of that paid for by Big Tobacco) was in consensus
on both the hazards of tobacco use and the efficacy of tax-induced price increases on youth smoking. They needed health policy and economic experts to
help craft a medically and economically sound reform plan, to validate it with
academic gravitas, and to defend it against the formidably credentialed experts of the insurers, free-market economists, and other threatened interests
who would challenge it. The campaign's experts would also reassure skeptical
legislators and citizens who remembered all too well the fate of the Clinton
health-care initiative.

Johns Hopkins University occupies a unique place in Maryland's con-
sciousness and its politics. Its credentialed faculty members often weigh in
on public discourse, and the university's voice is respected in Annapolis. In
no field is this truer than in public health. A connected Hopkins graduate,
DeMarco had a long history of seeking scientific support—and political ballast—from the Bloomberg School of Public Health at Johns Hopkins, beginning with his gun wars. In particular, he had built a strong relationship with

then dean Alfred Sommer, "an inspiration and a great help." After Beilenson recruited him, DeMarco says, "Sommer was the first person I wanted to go see about health-care reform." He and Beilenson had lunch with the dean, whom DeMarco describes as "very much an 'Okay, let's do it' kind of person. And he said, 'Okay, you need help devising a plan. We've got experts here; let's bring you and them together.'"

Sommer proceeded to do what DeMarco's campaigns thrive on: network. He connected DeMarco and Beilenson with health policy scholars throughout the Bloomberg School, five of whom, says DeMarco, "became the core of our expertise—Jonathan Weiner, Laura Morlock, Tom Oliver, Hugh Waters, Darrell Gaskin, along with Dean Diane Hoffman of the Maryland School of Law." Then this campaign would do something that social justice advocates rarely do: instead of the experts lecturing people about what they *should* want, they would listen to what people *did*, and *did not*, want.

Never Too Early for the Media Launch

Even though the campaign had not yet developed its concrete policy objectives, it was time for the next stage in this campaign: public education through the media. The goal was to convince Marylanders that change was both urgently needed and politically possible, beliefs essential as preconditions for any successful universal health-care campaign, no matter its details.

As in DeMarco's earlier campaigns, the coalition building and the public education efforts were mutually reinforcing, and each depended heavily on media coverage. "We have the habit of launching our campaign a thousand times, so that people finally take notice," Glenn Schneider notes. From the very first step that DeMarco and Beilenson took after they had funds in hand—the initial poll—they began talking to media gatekeepers. On August 12, 1999, they released the poll results. Although not a formal campaign launch, this was still the first call—and the first supporting evidence—for state health-care reform. And even though the poll was the news, the *Baltimore Sun* headline was "Md. Group Pushes for Health Reform."

By September, two new organizations were in place. The 501(c)(3) Maryland Citizens' Health Initiative Education Fund, Inc., would be free to take—wherever it could get it—apolitical philanthropic foundation money. And the 501(c)(4) Maryland Citizens' Health Initiative, Inc., could raise and spend nonpartisan election and lobbying money. DeMarco would be the executive director of both organizations, and Beilenson would chair both boards.

On October 4, 1999, the Maryland Citizens' Health Initiative formally launched the campaign. Though the tactical target dates lay far ahead—the

2002 elections and the 2003 legislative session—the vow to mobilize a phalanx of citizen groups was news enough. The *Sun* carried a long, prominent story, headlined "Maryland Ranks Near Top in Growth of Uninsured" above the subhead "Maryland Coalition Decries Rising Number of Uninsured." A broad-based coalition of community leaders, the *Sun* reported, had introduced a "Declaration of Health Care Independence" calling for quality affordable health care for all Marylanders.

DeMarco was already on the road drumming up media attention. Under the headline "Health Care Effort Looks to Students; Wilde Lake Visitor Targets High Schools for Support of Insurance Plan," the suburban Howard County edition of the October 4 *Sun* reported: "First it was gun safety, then curbing tobacco sales. Yesterday, Vincent DeMarco was back at Wilde Lake High School in Columbia for a third time, trying to recruit student support for his latest cause: universal health care for Maryland in 2003." From here on, the campaign's media coverage would, in its creativity, redundancy, relentlessness, and success, mirror the coverage of the cigarette tax campaign.

The Biggest Coalition Yet

By the end of 1999, Glenn Schneider and Rosanna Miles were helping DeMarco staff and organize the new Maryland Citizens' Health Initiative, and DeMarco began to envision a coalition whose size would dwarf that mobilized for the tobacco tax campaign or any citizen campaign. Yet at a meeting of 150 people early in 2000, Schneider became progressively uneasy: "People were signing lists; people were trying to recruit more people; we really couldn't fit a lot more folks in and get business done." At that point, Schneider says, he and DeMarco told the meeting about "this other organizing model, where we get organizations on board, and then we get the membership on board after that." Peter Beilenson said he thought that made sense, and then "Peter's deputy city health commissioner spoke up and suggested, 'Why don't we say our goal is two thousand groups?'"

Schneider was nonplussed. "I don't quite understand what you're talking about. Two thousand groups?" The deputy commissioner explained his thinking: "You got three hundred and fifty-some groups for the Children's Initiative. This is a much bigger project, so I would assume we need a lot more groups." Schneider agreed they needed more groups but suggested that "this two thousand thing is a little bit silly" and reminded the deputy commissioner, "*You* aren't going to be doing the phone calls."

The advocate was adamant: "Two thousand it is; it sounds great!" Schneider says he thought, "All right, let's stop here, let's talk about this. At the very least, let's chat, because this is a lot." But, finally, Schneider says: "We all just said, 'All right, we'll give it a shot. Hopefully, the media won't catch on too much that one of the big goals we have is an impossible two thousand groups.'" Meanwhile, Beilenson and DeMarco didn't yet know exactly what legislation they would seek. They hadn't designed the crucial organizing resolution they would ask potential coalition members to sign, mainly because they hadn't figured out how to craft a goal that could attract signatures from both single-payer and anything-but-single-payer advocates.

How were they going to get two thousand groups to come on board? Schneider describes the resolution they came up with, which "basically said, 'Would you agree that everyone has the right to have health care? Would you agree that physicians should get paid the amount that they deserve? That you should have total choice of physicians?' It was Mom and apple pie. It went with what our poll showed us as being the way to go, and it satisfied the single-payer people, too."

By the summer of 2000, DeMarco, Glenn Schneider, and Rosanna Miles had begun the climb toward two thousand groups, ignoring everything else that was going on, including in the legislature. Their strategy was simple and familiar, Schneider says: "Call, call, call, call, call!" He used his phone list from Smoke Free Maryland; Miles, her lists from the faith community; and DeMarco, his ever-expanding phone list—from Rolodex to smartphone—that went back to Young Democrats days.

During these months they discovered the magical organizing resource of energetic student interns. They drew upon highly motivated students from Johns Hopkins and the University of Maryland's medical and social work schools, who sometimes gained academic credit but always got invaluable on-the-ground experience. The interns brought not only fresh energy, but insight as well. One alert medical student uncovered a significant flaw in the team's recruitment strategy. While calling potential signatory organizations, he told Schneider, "I get kind of a weird response on the phone. It's because people don't know what in the world a Maryland Citizens' Health Initiative is. Are we selling vaccines? Are we selling insurance?" What would he suggest instead, Schneider wanted to know. "I think we should say what we are, Maryland Health Care for All," said the intern. "That's how we should answer the phone. That's what we should put on our envelopes." Schneider took the idea to DeMarco, and Maryland Health Care for All! became the health initiative's public calling card for the next ten years.

By the middle of 2000, even with the students' help, the campaign had only around a thousand groups on board. As Schneider had feared, they were struggling to meet their goal. The first five hundred or so, he said, had been relatively easy because they were mostly veterans of DeMarco's earlier cam-

paigns. As Schneider came to understand: "When you're successful participating in such campaigns, you see the benefit of what you've done; you get
it in your blood. You realize how exciting it is, and you want to keep doing it
forever." But expanding beyond these groups proved a lot harder, Schneider
concedes: "You've got to build new relationships. You've got to move people
from not having any position on health care to having a position."

There are challenges that a campaign can usefully throw money at. In late
2000, DeMarco and Beilenson had persuaded the giant Kellogg Foundation
that the emerging campaign could be a model for other state health-care expansion efforts. Kellogg's grant of $175,000 dwarfed any previous support. The
campaign speedily recruited and hired ten part-time community organizers
from every corner of the state, who fanned out to their own communities to
recruit new signatory groups to the resolution. Four months later, at a boisterous party at the home of old friends of DeMarco's, with "live music and lots of
happy coalition partners," says Schneider, "we held a little ceremony where we
celebrated our campaign-tracking thermometer reaching two thousand. We
took pictures of all our organizers, went out to lunch—the whole nine yards."

A press release went out, launching the campaign once more, with fanfare
and coverage around the state announcing the signatures of the two thousand
groups. As if to rub the news in the faces of nervous health insurers and of
other interests vested in the present system, the June 1, 2001, *Baltimore Sun*
ran the story on the front page of its business section. The muted response of
the president of Maryland Business for Responsive Government, the health
insurer lobby, Robert O. C. "Rocky" Worcester: "Nobody can quarrel with
accessible quality health care ... but who's going to pay for this?"

Getting It Right—and Facing the Consequences

DeMarco could summarize the goal of Health Care for All! in six
words: "quality affordable health care for everyone." But the group's "Mom
and apple pie" organizing resolution had skirted the hard part, the plan that
would both reach their policy goal and unite all two thousand groups—or at
least get enough of them passionately committed to overcome the resistance
of the powerful interests that would oppose any change that threatened their
economic stake in the present system.

Just as critical, what plan would answer the genuine hard questions posed
by skeptical legislators—as well as the not-so-genuine but nagging lobbyist-
inspired questions? As early as the spring of 2000, well before the campaign
had signed up its first thousand groups, DeMarco as political strategist was

troubled. He and Beilenson knew that single-payer advocates were right that the system they favored would provide universality and cost containment, but what if they were wrong that no other system was economically feasible? Maryland Health Care for All! needed to find out. If there was another way, it would need the blessing of economic experts invulnerable to charges of skewing the numbers.

They found just such experts in a highly regarded and conservative Washington, D.C.–based economics research firm, the Lewin Group, whom they charged to "explore the expected costs and impacts of two alternative universal health care plans for Maryland." One was a single-payer plan; the other was a multipayer model that would give employers the option of providing coverage to their employees, but with no fewer benefits than the state-run public plan model provided (the direction DeMarco was leaning toward). The new costs under either plan would be borne not by premium increases, but by new taxes—on payrolls, personal income, tobacco, and alcohol—and by existing government programs such as Medicare and Medicaid.

When Maryland Health Care for All! released the Lewin Group report to the public on May 2, 2000, the result, crows Glenn Schneider, was "a huge success." The message the campaign framed, he said, was that "a study today revealed that universal health care is economically doable at the state level." The study demonstrated, to no one's surprise, that a single-payer system would provide both universal coverage and substantial cost savings. But it also demonstrated that a new reform plan designed by the Hopkins team to provide health care for all Marylanders within the framework of the existing health-care system—without threatening anyone's existing coverage—would not cost too much more than the existing system.

The media, however, heralded only the cost savings of the single-payer system. Almost buried in an enthusiastic story in Baltimore's business journal, the *Maryland Daily Record*, was the economic verdict on the "more flexible system" from Hopkins: costs would rise "only" $207 million, the study's authors said. "Our single-payer friends," said Schneider, "took this to mean only one thing: This study shows that you save money if you do single payer. That's all they heard. But we showed it was doable, no matter how you do it, at the state level."

Division

As even-handed as the Lewin Group report may have been, it brought no accord among the signatories to the Health Care for All! resolution. The single-payer advocates who formed the initial core of supporters remained adamant that single payer was the only moral solution. One of their groups, a local organization calling itself the Universal Health Care Action Network (not to be confused with the much more pragmatic national UHCAN organization), prepared an extensive brief for the campaign that concluded: "Single-payer financed health care is the only means by which sufficient savings can be acquired to permit expansion of health care delivery with respect to both universality and comprehension. Universality is a moral imperative.... Any scheme that retains multi-payer, for-profit health care delivery cannot possibly save the money necessary to expand health care coverage without increasing costs." (In the meantime, the centrist Democratic Progressive Policy Institute was advising presidential candidate Al Gore to avoid even a whisper of single-payer advocacy, yet also to scorn the greedy Republican insurance industry alliance around the mythical power of the free market to do nothing but good.)

In Maryland, the opponents of any change at all in the system were already mobilizing. A former Baltimore delegate to the General Assembly, Dennis C. McCoy, now a State House lobbyist, had written to an army of potential opponents to whatever plan Beilenson and DeMarco came up with. Quoted by the *Baltimore Sun*'s Thomas W. Waldron on September 26, 2000, McCoy's call to arms got straight to the point: "We have identified your organization or some of your clients as having a direct interest in opposing socialized medicine and the efforts of Vinnie DeMarco to introduce this failed proposal into Maryland."

On September 25, 2000, McCoy convened a meeting of those who responded to the alarm, raising the specter of a DeMarco-inspired political juggernaut. The DeMarco team had caught wind of this meeting in time to have Bart Naylor, an old friend of DeMarco's and an economic consultant to Maryland Health Care for All!, slip in under McCoy's radar as the head of a nondescript consulting firm. There was much terrifying talk, says Naylor, about "this Vinny guy who is coming together with this plan, and it's a very dangerous idea." Naylor listened while McCoy warned his audience, "If the opponents stand divided, the legislature could easily get stampeded into doing something bad."

No one at the meeting knew Naylor, who kept pressing McCoy politely but firmly on exactly who was funding this convocation. Naylor reported that McCoy dodged the question, but "who" was not exactly a mystery. As the *Sun*'s Waldron wrote: "Some observers contend that DeMarco should be thrilled with opposition from McCoy, whose client list includes 'black hats' such as tobacco, casino and liquor companies. 'That's great—liquor, gambling, and tobacco leading the charge against health care for poor people,' said a lobbyist familiar with the issue."

Black hats or not, the aroused opposition was organizing—and refining the themes it would use to plague DeMarco's team. By November 17, 2000, the Montgomery County *Gazette* reported, it had formed a coalition and invited key legislative leaders to a briefing on "a practical and realistic approach to health care reform in Maryland," but it was hard to find in their diatribes any ideas that fit this description. Whatever plan Health Care for All! was about to develop, the opposition thundered, it would be "socialized health care"—a label that had sounded the death knell for generations of health-care plans. The *Gazette*'s Walter Lee Dozler reported that at this meeting, Thomas J. DiLorenzo, a conservative, credentialed expert in business and management at Maryland's Loyola College, "called the Maryland Citizens' Health Initiative an ideological special interest group that advocates socialized medicine" and said that if it succeeded, "health care would become more costly and many of the best and brightest medical professionals would leave to work in states where they could earn market-rate salaries." Furthermore, he contended, "everyone already gets health care in Maryland. They may be without health insurance, but everyone gets health care."

Others at the briefing reported on by the *Gazette* claimed that the single-payer model was economically unfeasible, pointing at the (fictionally) failing national health-care systems in Canada and Great Britain. A spokesperson for the benignly named Council for Affordable Health Insurance, the Maryland health insurers' own lobby, offered details, as the *Gazette* story reported: "As we have seen in other countries that have universal care, services will become rationed. In Canada, where they have universal health care, they have only a handful of MRI machines in the whole country. People will not be able to gain the medical attention they need." Such arguments impressed at least one key legislator at the meeting, Democratic House Speaker Casper Taylor, whose suggestion revealed his position: "Let's analyze the single-payer system and prove to ourselves why it doesn't work."

In other settings, legislators were asking hard questions. In his September 26 article, the *Sun*'s Waldron quoted one delegate from Baltimore County who wanted to know: "What happens when we run out of money? We'll either have to raise taxes or people will do without health care." He quoted another who argued that universal health care could not be implemented state by state; if it were, Maryland "would become a dumping ground for every sick person in the Mid-Atlantic region." Such incredulity by legislators confirmed DeMarco's caution in staying away from the legislature until a concrete health-care plan could be put forward that would answer such questions.

The Rule of the Thirds

How would DeMarco and Beilenson slash through this thicket of conflicting visions? By the fall of 2000, it was becoming clear to both men that Maryland Health Care for All! would fail if it proposed a single-payer plan. They knew they had to discuss this as soon as possible with the single-payer advocates in the coalition, so they called a meeting for mid-November that DeMarco calls "one of the hardest I ever had to preside over."

> I tried to explain what I had learned from polling and talking with people around the state—that Marylanders would just not accept being taken off their health insurance plans to be put on one government-run plan. Peter described how impractical it was to try single payer at the state level when so many federal waivers would be needed which would be almost impossible to get.
>
> The single-payer people lost their minds. They denounced us for betraying the cause. They said that any health-care expansion or health care for all plan which was not single payer was not worth doing. In fact, they argued that it was a mistake to expand Medicaid to poor people because it would reduce the societal pressure for single payer.
>
> This is where I had had enough of the single-payer-or-nothing crowd. To me, it was just wrong not to try to expand health-care access for those who desperately needed it by the means we have available in order to build support for the ultimate single-payer panacea.

DeMarco had encountered the conundrum that so many social justice campaigns face: the clash between those who see the good as the enemy of the best, and those who, like DeMarco, see significant incremental change as far preferable to a near certain dead-end campaign. Speaking of dead-end campaigns, he cites a haunting analogy: "What especially outraged me was that these were the very same people who had just elected George W. Bush president by voting for Ralph Nader in the 2000 presidential election."

After the meeting, the office started getting calls from one-time supporters and colleagues, single-payer advocates, who "all of a sudden," Schneider says, "were saying nasty things about what we were doing." Less rigid members of the single-payer community, like Health Care for the Homeless, may not have liked the decision but understood it. About 40 percent of those who had come to the early meetings were "diehards," Schneider says, unwilling to compromise.

Nothing induces more pain in a campaign strategist/leader than perceiving a need to compromise—to accept less than the full campaign objective and, if so, how much less? A coalition, especially a DeMarco coalition, is painstakingly built to support a specific, concrete objective that speaks to the priorities of each segment of the coalition; this is the glue that holds the coalition together. Pulling back any element of the objective thus threatens, at worst, the participation, at best the fervor, of the coalition members who had bargained for just that element.

This is also where the ideal confronts the pragmatic, and the subterranean schism between idealists and pragmatists surfaces. True believers like the single-payer advocates have a hard time hearing the idea that making any significant advance in the foreseeable future demands that compromises be made now. As Bishop Miles commented:

> The single-payer people don't live in the world as it is. They live in the world as it should be. And when you live in the world as it should be, solely, then you become irrelevant. I think that's what's happened to single payers, that they become irrelevant to the argument. Good politics is the ability to compromise. And if you can't strike that balance, then you soon become irrelevant to the issues of the day.
>
> I think it was Martin Luther King who said if you love without power, it's sentimental, and power without love is crass. You need to be able to strike the balance. You need your zealots to keep you reminded that what you are ultimately aiming for is the world as it should be and to move the world as it is in that direction. But understand that you don't achieve that overnight. And many times it's baby steps that you take.

Glenn Schneider puts the decision to abandon pursuit of a single-payer system in a strategic axiom that he and DeMarco have developed during the years they have campaigned together. They call it the Rule of the Thirds:

> During the Maryland Children's Initiative campaign, Vinny and I decided to travel down to the lower Shore area to attend the annual Tawes Crab and Clam Bake—an annual feast of crab and politics where every political who-ha showed each year. It was a two- to three-hour master class for me given that the event predated the arrival of mobile e-mails. Vinny did talk a lot on his cell phone but we also got a lot of talking in. . . .
>
> On the way, we discussed and developed further what we called the Rule of the Thirds. If you gauge public support for any public health campaign, you could split it up as follows:
>
> The *Rabid Third* of the population are those who deeply support your campaign. They will do anything: show up for rallies, help stuff envelopes, give money, recruit others. They care big time about what you are doing.

A typical statement of Rabid Thirds: "I will do whatever I can to help you. I don't have much time or money to give but whatever I have, it's yours. Thanks for doing this. It means a lot to me."

The *Middle Third* of the population are those who support your campaign. They self-identify with what you are doing. *But* when you ask them to do things, they may have other more important things scheduled. They may be willing to call their lawmakers for you but are not so hot on the rally idea. Money might be a hard thing to extract. But they still think your campaign's a good idea. A typical statement of Middle Thirds: "I am so glad that *you* are out there doing this. This is a really important thing for you to do. Let me know what I can do to help and I'll try to fit it in."

The *Anti-Third* of the population hate your campaign and everything about it. They identify with your opponents and will either be deeply opposed, where they will actively give time, talent, and treasure to your opponents, *or* they will just be mildly opposed and do absolutely nothing. A typical statement of Anti-Thirds: "This is government at its worst. You are taking away our freedoms, blah, blah, blah."

So the big two questions that you might ask: (1) Who should I try to recruit? and (2) Where can I find that population? Most people say, "Recruit the Middle Third and try to change them into Rabids." Actually, it's the Rabid Third that you try to recruit. They are the ones who will do anything for your cause. They care deeply about it and will do their best to see you through to victory.

Also, we've found that most people do not change from a Middle to a Rabid unless something deeply personal inspires a conversion (for example, losing someone to tobacco use, quitting smoking after many attempts, et cetera).

You can find the Rabid Thirds in every organization you try to recruit. They self-select and if you pay attention, you'll find them. After a big talk, they might say things like, "What you said really hit home. I want to help and here's my story." They might as well have a Rabid Third T-shirt on. If we properly target the right groups to recruit to our coalition, we may find a bunch of Rabid Thirds all at once.

This goes back to why we picked a $1.50 tax for our MCI campaign or health care for all for our health care goal. Issue goal selection is critical. It must inspire the Rabid Thirds. They must really get juiced about it. That's why Smoke Free Maryland did not want to move on the dime tax offered to us the year before we started the MCI campaign. It did not move any of the diehards. Who wants to fight for a dime when perhaps we can get a dollar if we wait a year?

But the issue picked must still be acceptable to the Middle Third. Though they won't do a lot to tangibly support you, they still have to think what you've proposed is reasonable. In all our campaigns, polling showed we hit the mark with our campaign selection.

If we had gone with the single-payer idealists, we would have gained and kept a very Rabid Third. But we would have *lost* the Middle Third. You have to excite the Rabids and keep the Middles supporting your work. That's the balance required. [Even as this is written, in the summer of 2009, with health-care reform at the top of the national agenda, a new poll by Celinda Lake finds that when asked to choose between DeMarco's health care for all plan, which builds on the present system, and a single-payer plan, voters chose the health care for all plan by 64 percent to 18 percent.]

The drift away from a single-payer plan became public knowledge with a December 20, 2000, article in the *Sun* headlined, "Single-Payer Quest Abandoned." On behalf of Maryland Health Care for All!, Beilenson announced: "We've come to the conclusion the single-payer is basically unfeasible in a Bush Administration.... Pragmatically, the best way is to look at a multipayer option." The article quoted the jubilant Rocky Worcester, who spoke for the health insurer lobby, Maryland Business for Responsive Government, boasting that his group was "happy with the effect we've had in bringing this back to the center." Worcester also conceded that the number of uninsured in Maryland was a problem. DeMarco seized upon Worcester's statement, claiming that "change in the dialogue already marked a success for his group which was launched just a year ago. 'The question has changed from whether we have health care for all Marylanders to how.'"

Still Listening

Between January and June 2001, Maryland Health Care for All! held eleven town meetings in churches, community centers, colleges, and high schools, drawing 742 Maryland residents—325 from rural counties and 417 from urban or suburban counties. Most of those who testified did so on the part of organizations, churches, unions, and civic groups representative of thousands of Marylanders. "I think this is one of the really key things we did," says DeMarco, "to bring together the stakeholders, the people, and the experts, to learn from each other and help the experts come up with a plan that made sense for Maryland."

For the first time, Glenn Schneider said, "we were talking about health care in the state, and we had a hundred people in a room. Whether it be Baltimore City or in western Maryland or on the Eastern Shore, people were coming because they cared about the issue enough to give their opinion to these experts that were in the room who wanted to form a plan based on their opinion."

The citizens of Maryland told the experts the same things DeMarco had heard in his travels around the state: Yes, people generally supported extending health care to the uninsured. But if they had health insurance themselves, they wanted the option to keep it and not to be forced into a government plan with all the uninsured. They mostly opposed scrapping the current system for a government-run system. Instead, they favored expanding what was good in the present system and getting rid of what was bad. Few of the faith groups, civic groups, unions, and other advocacy groups that had been essential to DeMarco's earlier coalitions were ready to support a single-payer system. Neither were any of the stakeholders, from doctors and nurses to government regulators, convened in small groups where they could feel free to air their needs and fears.

After Two Years, a Draft Plan

There is a reflexive aversion among many grassroots activists to academic experts (and, indeed, credentialed experts of any kind). They perceive these ivory tower dwellers as insensitive to the daily lives and concerns of the people and issues they purport to be expert about. DeMarco did not let that happen between the concerned citizens, the stakeholders, and the Hopkins experts. "At some point," says Schneider, "there was a real conversion of the experts, from 'We are your paid experts' to 'We are a part of this great moving coalition, and we want to come up with the best plan we can. And we are here with you.'"

In the spring and summer of 2001, with a timely grant from The Robert Wood Johnson Foundation and under the leadership of Dean Sommer and health policy scholar Jonathan Weiner, Johns Hopkins formally convened a panel of experts in health-care policy, public health policy, economics, and law to integrate the feedback from the stakeholder and town meetings and to develop a draft legislative plan. By September, the panel had finalized the details of their plan, but not without constant feedback from DeMarco and Schneider, always with an ear to the sensitivities of the public, as well as the concerns of the groups that needed to be kept aboard the campaign.

On the night of September 5, Schneider was in the office with DeMarco fine-tuning the plan the experts had come up with. "It's 11:30, and Vinny says, 'Do you mind if I go home right now? I have a half an hour left of my wedding anniversary.' I said, 'I know, Vinny, I'm so sorry.' So he went home. I left, eventually, at 3 or 3:30, and we announced the plan the next day, to a lot of fanfare."

The draft plan went out to each of the more than twenty-one hundred Health Care for All! groups. "The document that you are about to read is the most comprehensive and complete proposal for universal health reform ever developed in Maryland's history," Dean Sommer wrote in the introduction. "It is also one of the most comprehensive blueprints for state-level reform ever crafted anywhere in this nation."

At this juncture, DeMarco and Beilenson faced a dual challenge: they needed to encapsulate the plan in legislative language and, simultaneously, to maintain the cohesion and energy of a coalition that had waited nearly two years for a concrete legislative objective, now peppered with passionate single-payer outliers who were sullen and, in some cases, mutinous.

From September to November 2001, the educational arm of Maryland Health Care for All!—the Maryland Citizens' Health Initiative Education Fund (safe for foundations to fund)—organized thirteen more town meetings around Maryland. The stated intent of these meetings of coalition members and the concerned public was to review the draft legislative proposal, answer questions, and solicit feedback. The pragmatic intent was to transform the support of the original signers for the broad, vague resolution into support for the concrete plan. Simultaneously, the staff fanned out to brief key coalition organizations. In the hundreds of comments they got back from the coalition, it became clear to DeMarco "that there were things in our draft plan that were not going to fly." With the help of the Hopkins team and Michael Miller of Boston-based Community Catalyst, a national nonprofit that works for strengthening the health-care system, they analyzed the comments, and the plan was tweaked until DeMarco was convinced it would satisfy the key organizations in the coalition.

A Canny Strategy—or Foot Dragging?

As 2002 approached, members of Maryland Health Care for All! argued over when to release their final plan. Some coalition members pressed for a 2002 release and for making the plan an issue in the 2002 elections. DeMarco was certain this would not work: "We hadn't really educated the public, and certainly our policymakers, on some of the key elements, such as requiring businesses to chip in a fair-share piece of it." The plan's most formidable political hurdle, and the essence of its financial viability, was a mandate that required all employers, large or small, either to provide health-care coverage at prescribed minimum standards, or to contribute the equivalent to a state fund for the uninsured. The coalition decided to keep working on the plan, with a target release date of December 2002, after its critical ally Kathleen Kennedy Townsend presumably had been elected governor.

Meanwhile, to rally coalition members restive for action, the DeMarco team developed a second campaign track: a modest but appealing agenda that could serve as a strong foundation for a candidate pledge campaign in the 2002 state elections. "We knew we needed a new resolution," Glenn Schneider says, "and we thought, what do we need, how can we do this? Let's talk about something for people who have insurance."

That "something" turned out to be an issue on the near horizon that threatened a steep rise in health insurance rates for those who relied for their insurance on the state's largest health insurer, CareFirst, the Maryland Blue Cross Blue Shield agency. While a wave of buy-outs by for-profit insurance companies was engulfing other state Blue Cross insurers, CareFirst had remained a nonprofit organization. But now, it faced a buy-out. "We had to think about stopping that," Schneider says, "because all of our national friends warned us, if they go for-profit, they raise prices, they cut benefits." The Health Care for All! Board, and particularly prominent Maryland labor leader Ernie Crofoot, strongly backed including in the resolution support for keeping CareFirst nonprofit.

The team then decided to pursue a single element that they knew would have to be incorporated in their final plan: raising the cigarette tax. They would aim for thirty-six cents, capturing the last installment of the dollar increase they had campaigned for since 1997, and the increase would go toward expanding health-care coverage. Next, they looked for an objective that would engage senior citizens, as both a population at risk and an essential force in the coalition; they chose making prescription drugs more affordable.

Now they had a package to take to itchy coalition members. As Schneider summarizes it: "Will you help us work to get health care for all, and support these three policy initiatives? Keeping Blue Cross Blue Shield a nonprofit; a tobacco tax for health care; and reducing prescription drug costs for seniors by creating a buying pool."

A "Freedom Summer": Recharging the Campaign

How could a handful of staff members and interns reach out quickly but respectfully to all twenty-two hundred groups that had signed the first resolution, to ask them instead to sign a less ambitious one? Schneider hit on an idea inspired by Laura Morlock, one of the Hopkins experts. She had told him that the reason she cared so much about movements like this was because of her experience as a student during the 1964 Mississippi "Freedom Summer" civil rights movement. "I thought, 'Health care is a civil rights issue.' Wouldn't that be neat if we could do the same thing?"

DeMarco and Schneider planned two pushes for the summer of 2002, as the election campaigns heated up for fall. They needed to go out and talk to all twenty-two hundred groups and get them to sign on to the new three-point resolution, and they needed to canvas in key areas around the state to encourage individual families to also sign on to the resolution. Where would the students for their own Freedom Summer come from? The leadership of the American Medical Student Association based in Virginia stepped up and, Schneider says, responded, "Oh, that's a great idea!" Sixty-five students signed up, and "some actually traveled, staying with relatives, and some folks came for the whole summer, found a job here, found somewhere to live, so they could spend their whole summer with us. So we had this amazing summer, where we had all these students coming, doing all this canvassing work, and seventeen hundred organizations signed the pledge, thirty-eight hundred families signed on."

The campaign had gained momentum. The number of engaged groups, more than seventeen hundred, was almost as intimidating as the twenty-two hundred that had signed the original resolution. There were concrete legislative objectives to *keep* the coalition members engaged through the 2002 legislative assembly. The package of policy initiatives in the new resolution could become the basis for a candidate pledge campaign in the 2002 elections in the summer and fall—and the initiatives would help separate candidates who were open to expanding health care for all from candidates who were resistant. Above all, the stage would be set for a Townsend governorship, and action on the comprehensive bill.

8

Follow the Leaders,
Lead the Leaders

From 1999 through 2002, as DeMarco and Beilenson developed their Health Care for All! plan, DeMarco was paying at least as much attention to the legislative environment that plan would face as to the polls, the consultations, the Hopkins experts, and the media. Although the chairs of the key committees that would handle health-care legislation would be important players in the plan's legislative success, the fate of most legislation rests in the hands of the three great Maryland power holders: the governor, the speaker of the House, and the Senate president. Who would they be after 2002, and above all, who would be governor?

The DeMarco team was certain that powerful, sympathetic inside leadership lay just around the corner in the person of Lieutenant Governor Kathleen Kennedy Townsend. Maryland's term limit law would end Governor Glendening's tenure, and the popular Townsend, enhanced by the historic aura of her father, Robert Kennedy, was the odds-on favorite to be elected to succeed him. This was grounds for optimism: DeMarco was closer, philosophically, politically, and personally, to Townsend than to Glendening. Her anticipated ascendancy colored all his planning.

At critical points in DeMarco's campaigns, Townsend had been there— serving as the centerpiece for rallies, helping with fund-raising, writing supportive op-ed pieces, and lobbying quietly but hard. During the 2002 elections, because of the Maryland Citizens' Health Initiative nonprofit legal status, there could be no overt coordination between that effort and the Townsend campaign, but there could be felicitous synergy. There could be a vigorous, nonpartisan election campaign to make voters aware of just which gubernatorial candidates were supportive of health care for all and which were not. Almost all of those opposed would be Republicans, especially the conservative Republican candidate, Robert Ehrlich.

On July 10, the *Sun* headlined: "Coalition Unveils Health Care Pledge." The pledge mirrored the latest coalition-organizing resolution, calling upon candidates for governor to sign on the line to support a thirty-six-cent cigarette tax increase for expanded health-care coverage, to stop the sale of the nonprofit CareFirst health insurer to a for-profit buyer, and to authorize the state to negotiate lower drug prices. Simultaneous with the pledge campaign launch, Health Care for All! released a new poll showing that Maryland voters strongly supported all three measures.

Townsend signed the pledge. Her opponent, Ehrlich, said: "We are pro-business. Therefore, we will not be signing this." By September 12, the Interdenominational Ministerial Alliance was running a new version of the "Bang! Cough! Ka-ching!" ad, substituting this year's villain, Ehrlich, for the last campaign's villain, Ellen Sauerbrey, as the tool of the gun, tobacco, and casino lobbies. Regarding Ehrlich, nonpartisan DeMarco told the *Sun*: "Where Kathleen endorsed the tobacco tax, he's taken $30,000 in contributions from tobacco companies." This proved to be, as DeMarco lamented, "the only hit" that Ehrlich took during the campaign. Not only was 2002 a Republican year throughout the country, but also Townsend's campaign fell short. DeMarco's political eulogy: "She's a wonderful person who would have made a great governor."

In the wake of the election, on November 12, *Sun* political commentator Howard Libit and reporter David Nitkin had the last word on the pledge campaign as they tallied up the election's winners and losers: "Vincent DeMarco: Devoted to progressive politics, he saw his entire agenda go down the drain. Townsend signed DeMarco's 'Health Care for All' pledge backing a thirty-six-cent tobacco tax increase. Ehrlich didn't. Townsend promised tougher gun laws that DeMarco, an anti-handgun advocate, also supported. Ehrlich said he'd review the gun laws to see if some should go. DeMarco has had notable success in the past, but the next four years could be his toughest."

Grieving

According to Schneider, Townsend's defeat felt like the undoing of the whole campaign:

Vinny had been down at the headquarters to celebrate. It's probably the only night of the year when Vinny stays up past midnight. It's kind of like his own Christmas. This was where you saw the fruits of your labor; after working on the election for months and months, this was where you got to see what happened. I had a sense of dread going into that evening. I would spend the first few hours with our local Democratic campaign headquarters; I just remember sitting there watching results come in. It soon became very clear that we were going to have an awful night gubernatorially. I was sitting there watching the results come in, and then the whole party shut down early. I went home. Clearly, they were devastated down at the headquarters, too, and Vinny went home early that night too.

I remember thinking, "What does this mean to our overall campaign?" There was a sense of loss, a real pivotal grieving point. The following few days in the office were really hard. Vinny hardly came in. We were here, but we weren't really here. We were trying to figure out how to couch this for our coalition. We always put out e-mails to give our coalition members a sense of where we were in our campaign. And it was usually my job to come up with something. I just remember thinking, "I'm not exactly sure how or what we're going to do to make this seem like a positive event."

I said to Vinny, "Well, what about the campaign?" And he said, "I'm just not sure if anything can be done now." I said, "But we can't just quit. Vinny, there's a lot of people depending on us." I actually felt a sense of abandonment. We even got to the point where Vinny thought about how he could make a graceful exit. He said, "Glenn, this could be your chance." And I said, "I don't want this to be my chance. This is not what I foresaw happening. And quite honestly, we need you. I don't want you to leave."

As DeMarco surveyed the new legislative environment, though, his optimism slowly rekindled. He would not quit. The Republicans had overreached in their fantasy that they could significantly cut into the Democrats' control of the legislature. The Democrats kept their overwhelming margins in both houses, and seventy House delegates, just short of a seventy-one House majority, and eighteen of the twenty-four senators needed for a Senate majority had signed the Health Care for All! pledge. "You know, it wasn't such a disastrous election," DeMarco says now.

One apparent disaster turned out to be anything but. "The Republicans felt they had done two great things," DeMarco explains. "They had elected the first governor in thirty years and defeated the Democratic speaker of the House, Casper Taylor, which sent shockwaves everywhere." A conservative Democrat—Taylor had opposed the tobacco tax in 1999—he had held a constraining grip on a far more liberal House membership. "The consequence," says DeMarco, "was that Mike Busch became speaker. They just did not at all think that the consequence was going to be a very progressive new speaker. The Republicans came to regret that so much."

All 140 of Busch's colleagues voted to elect him, and he still served as speaker in 2009. Deeply respected, he is also a formidable figure, courted as a tackle in college by the National Football League until a knee injury ended his playing career. Before his ascendancy to speaker, he served for many years as chair of the House Economic Matters Committee, where he led success-ful legislative initiatives on health care and education funding. In 2000 and 2001, he had sponsored and headed efforts to make prescription drugs more affordable and accessible for seniors and low-income individuals, and, since 2002, he had been fighting to keep CareFirst from converting to a for-profit company—two issues the new Health Care for All! pledge supported.

Busch was a natural leader for DeMarco to work with and to follow. But first, DeMarco had to overcome a not insignificant hurdle. Recall that DeMarco had decided not to push health-care expansion in the previous leg-islative assembly session in 2002. Yet Busch, as chair of the Economic Matters Committee, was then pressing hard for health care measures of his own. The restlessness that embroiled DeMarco's decision to wait among many of the most impatient Health Care for All! Coalition members paled in comparison with the acute frustration of Mike Busch. DeMarco shudders at the memory: "Mike Busch was very unhappy that we were doing all this work and not talk-ing to his committee. I'll never forget this: In 2002, he called me before his committee in public and just reamed me out, up and down, about how ri-diculous it was that we were out there talking to people about these grandiose plans while he had all these health-care bills before his committee that had an impact or could have an impact." He demanded to know why DeMarco hadn't appeared before his committee, testifying for and against the bills.

In front of the committee, DeMarco had explained that they were "trying to talk to people for a while and come back to you when we have a coalition and we have a plan." Busch's response: "We got things going on right here, right now, Mr. DeMarco—we need help." Behind the scenes, DeMarco told Busch that the Maryland Citizens' Health Initiative was a 501(c)(3) organiza-tion and was restricted in how much lobbying it could do. That explanation didn't fly either. "I took a real shellacking," DeMarco says. "But I think that helped Busch get that out of his system." Time, and DeMarco's persistence, would heal the breach. In the meantime, as speaker, Busch created a new House Health and Government Operations Committee with a strong, commit-ted chair, John Hurson, an attorney from liberal Montgomery County and a longtime ally of DeMarco's.

The Chameleon Campaign

Until the defeat of Kathleen Kennedy Townsend, DeMarco had fol-lowed the essential elements of his strategic template: media advocacy, or-ganizing, trial run, and the elections. Townsend's loss and the election of a sworn opponent to the goals of Health Care for All! threw a wrench into the template's workings. Yet with unwavering support from Peter Beilenson and the Health Care for All! Board, most of whose members had been with DeMarco for years of campaigning, DeMarco stuck with it. They would continue publicly to advocate their comprehensive plan just as if Townsend had won, although internally they were reconciled to reality: this plan would have to remain an unattainable goal as long as Ehrlich was governor. The key to meeting the challenge of their new circumstances would be finding common ground with the remaining supportive leaders within the legislature; circumventing, wherever possible, the governor's power; and seizing new opportunities that might arise as unexpectedly as Townsend's defeat.

On December 9, 2002, the Maryland Citizens' Health Initiative released its plan for universal health care for all Marylanders. The December 10 *Baltimore Sun* article by William Salganik is briefed in the *Sun*'s archive: "Plan unveiled to buy health care for uninsured; Guaranteed health-coverage plan unveiled; Firms not offering benefit would pay into a fund. Plan to buy health care for uninsured unveiled. Md. legislative package would provide coverage to 500,000, bolster local clinics."

The messenger was the leader of the Johns Hopkins team, Jonathan Weiner, professor of health policy and management, who promised, "Maryland can be a leader with this private-oriented initiative." But even the new lobbyist for Health Care for All!, Sean Cavanaugh, was candid about their plans and the chances in the 2003 session, which would be dominated by a record budget deficit—no time for an increase in health-care funding. The session would also be the first test of strength between a new Republican governor in a constitutionally strong role and a Democratic legislature used to having its own way. "It's certainly not going to pass this year," Cavanaugh acknowledged, "but we can do a lot of education." And DeMarco, Schneider, and Miles went to work again, getting hundreds of groups to sign a new health care for all resolution.

The predictions for nonaction in the 2003 legislative assembly proved more accurate than had the predictions that Townsend would become governor. The bill embodying the plan had sponsors in both legislative houses, and hearings, but "it went nowhere," says DeMarco; "no health care went anywhere." Nonetheless, Schneider insists that the 2003 session was "another great year." He pointed to more groups signing on to the final plan; more people getting the chance to testify before the House Health and Government Operations Committee, where the bill garnered eight votes of the thirteen needed to report it out of committee; and "good progress with the legislators who attended those hearings."

Nevertheless, Schneider knew as well as DeMarco that these modest vote gains on their grand health-care proposal, however close, would not be sufficient to keep up the spirit and energy of the Health Care for All! Coalition. They determined to pursue the set of lesser but substantial health-care objectives embraced by the candidate pledge and pressed by their new leadership support in the legislature, none of which would require the governor's signature.

First, they succeeded in squelching the for-profit sale of CareFirst, also a prime objective of Speaker Busch. The decision-making process began with the state insurance commissioner, a holdover from the Glendening administration. Then the legislature had ninety days within which it could override the commissioner's decision. The governor had no role to play. The Maryland Health Care for All! Coalition had been mobilized in late 2002 to bombard the commissioner with hearing testimony and letters from consumers; the labor, faith, and business communities; and physicians and other health-care professionals. The coalition's consultant, Bart Naylor, put together a strong brief arguing why CareFirst should stay not-for-profit. The insurance commissioner turned down the proposal to make CareFirst for-profit just after the start of the 2003 legislative session. The coalition then took the lead again, this time calling and writing legislators, urging them to let the commissioner's decision stand. Despite a fierce lobbying effort by the executives of CareFirst, inspired to frantic action by the prospect of $120 million in executive bonuses if the deal went through, the legislature, shepherded by the new health leadership, held firm.

This solid victory was just what the DeMarco team and the coalition needed. "On this," DeMarco says, "the single-payer people were all with us; everybody was united behind keeping CareFirst from being bought for a for-profit." Because of the coalition's weighty support on this issue, "a big change" took place in DeMarco's relationship with Mike Busch, who "has been absolutely wonderful on all the issues we work on." (It didn't hurt that DeMarco had hired lobbyist Sean Cavanaugh, who had worked closely with Busch in the past and continued to enjoy his trust.)

Next came a campaign to save prescription drug benefits, also out of the governor's reach. In early November 2003, the Maryland Health Care Commission, which mandates minimum health-care coverage for small employers, was under pressure from cost-cutting hawks in the Ehrlich administration to eliminate the prescription drug benefit from the state's Comprehensive Standard Health Benefit Plan. The Maryland Health Care for All! Coalition descended upon the commission hearings with a battery of impressive witnesses and besieged commission members with letters. The commission retained the prescription drug benefit.

Finally, to spare impoverished families a hike in insurance premiums, the coalition successfully mobilized to defeat an Ehrlich-backed bill that would have extended the child insurance premium of thirty-seven dollars a month for families earning 200 to 300 percent above the poverty line only to families earning 185 percent or less above the line. This campaign, too, resonated with the intent of the legislative Democratic leaders—even DeMarco's ofttimes adversary Senate President Miller—to challenge the polarizing new Republican governor.

In each of these successes the Health Care for All! Coalition redeemed DeMarco's vow, made to his campaign allies after he had recovered from the gloom of the Ehrlich election: "We want to go forward, not backward."

A Helping Hand from the Media

Despite DeMarco's positive turn of mind, he admits, after the legislative session ended in April 2003, the campaign's cause for being—universal health care—was going nowhere. "We had the coalition," DeMarco says, "we had a bill now, but it was hard to see the next step."

Then, in early June, "just out of the blue," DeMarco got a call from *Sun* reporter Julie Bell, partly because he was now known as a leading advocate of heath-care reform, but also as a result of his intense cultivation of the *Sun*'s journalists, including Bell, and his ability to help guide them to the significance of a story. Bell had called to tell him about an intriguing informal interview she had just had with Ehrlich's new health secretary, Nelson J. Sabatini. DeMarco's relationship with Sabatini, who had been health secretary for former Democratic governor William Donald Schaefer, "had never been positive. He thought I was some wacko guy." Did DeMarco know, the reporter asked now, that Sabatini says health care is a right, that Maryland should have universal health care—health care for all?

DeMarco asked where the secretary had said this. At a press conference? he asked, "with the governor standing by?" No, said the reporter, just in conversation with her. DeMarco went on to describe the Health Care for All! plan, which, he says, "helped make her story. She could say the secretary of health says everyone should have health care and there's a plan here how to do it." It took Bell's story appearing on the *Sun*'s front page on June 4 to make DeMarco realize its significance. It was headlined, "Top Administrator says Ehrlich Backs Concept of Universal Coverage." "That story was really like a match on a tinderbox," says DeMarco. By June 15, the ever alert *Sun* columnist Fraser Smith was on top of the story with a strong call for reform, under the headline, "State's Health Care Jalopy Needs a Major Tune-up."

The following day, June 16, the *Sun* ran an op-ed column signed by Beilenson and DeMarco (drafted by DeMarco and Schneider). It opened: "Maryland Health Secretary Nelson J. Sabatini recently issued a clarion call for universal health care in our state, and if Marylanders listen, we will all be healthier for it." The column reviewed the Health Care for All! plan, which nobody had paid any attention to since December "because of Ehrlich," DeMarco said. With the Sabatini story and the op-ed piece, "everybody who had been looking at us and not seeing us, saw us," as DeMarco puts it. "All of sudden, everybody in Maryland's talking about health care and coming to us for interviews that before we could never get." With those few words from Secretary Sabatini, said Glenn Schneider, "the world brightened. We resolved where we were going, and everything made sense."

Most important, the Sabatini quotation and the stories energized the legislative leadership. "Before," says DeMarco, "they were saying, 'How do we do that with Ehrlich there?' But now suddenly, Ehrlich's secretary of health is saying this. And then [House Health Committee and Government Operations chair] John Hurson called and said, 'Let's talk.'" DeMarco acknowledges that the primary force behind the movement toward health-care expansion lay with the key legislative leaders "who had wanted to do something on health care for a while. But they needed an opening, and the Sabatini remark opened the door for them and us in substantial ways." He describes the legislature's change of heart as a near epiphany. "Like you're looking at something all your life, but you don't see it. Suddenly, something sparks in your head, and you ask yourself, 'How come I never saw that before?' That is how Maryland legislators started viewing health-care expansion after the Sabatini remark and our follow-up. And it was wonderful."

The talk with Hurson led to a joint House/Senate Health Summit, convened in November by the leadership of both bodies: House Speaker Mike Busch, Senate President Mike Miller, and Senate Majority Leader Nathaniel J. McFadden, a Baltimore Democrat and DeMarco's own senator, who intended to introduce the Health Care for All! bill in the 2004 session. Saddled with his health secretary's acknowledgment of the need for health-care expansion, the governor, grudgingly, also agreed to cosponsor the summit.

In Maryland, DeMarco says, "there has never been anything like this before or since." Beilenson presented the Health Care for All! proposal to the roomful of legislators at the Health Summit, and "although it was clear that our whole proposal was not going to get enacted in 2004, all the legislative leaders said that they were committed to doing something substantial that year." Legislatively speaking, they "were definitely in the mix: the legislative health leaders were looking closely at our plan to see which parts of it could become part of a package that became law. And we were working with them to make sure that whatever they pushed through really helped to expand health care in Maryland. We went into the 2004 session feeling very hopeful about something good happening."

The 2004 Legislative Session

As the 2004 legislative session started, health-care reform legislation abounded, backed by the most powerful legislative leaders—even though, as the *Baltimore Sun*'s Salganik cautioned in his column of February 14, 2004, headed "Plan Unveiled to Provide Health Care for Uninsured," the expansion would come at a time "when most states, pressed for cash, are cutting back on their Medicaid programs; . . . 49 have cut Medicaid." Delegate Jim Hubbard in the House (who would always be the lead House sponsor) and Majority Leader McFadden in the Senate introduced the Health Care for All! plan, although it was not likely to pass, as DeMarco acknowledged, because of the powerful business opposition to its mandate that all state businesses either pay for in-suring their workers at a prescribed minimum percentage of their payroll or pay into a fund to cover the uninsured.

John Hurson, chair of the House Health and Government Operations Committee, introduced a health-care package that drew heavily on elements of the Health Initiative's bill. Included was a measure to extend to health maintenance organizations (HMOs) the 2 percent tax on premiums already being paid by other insurance companies, which would raise $50 million to be matched by Medicaid to expand health care to more than fifty thousand adults living below the federal poverty line. Hurson's bill would also have wid-ened the safety net for the uninsured by expanding state support for com-munity clinics. The bill was cosponsored in the Senate by the chairs of the two committees that handled health legislation. The Hurson bill and others also incorporated one provision dear to DeMarco's labor constituency: it would have required the state's largest businesses to allocate a specific percentage of their payroll for health care.

DeMarco's inside allies, in the right leadership roles and as strongly mo-tivated as they had ever been, matched in readiness his outside forces, whom DeMarco described to Salganik as a thousand organizations "chomping at the bit!" (DeMarco acknowledges that they had not secured the support of all those that had signed onto their earlier resolution: "We just did not have time to reach them all, but very few of them, like the single-payer groups, expressly said 'No' to the specific resolution.") Happily, 501(c)(3) foundation money was not in short supply, and 501(c)(4) political issue campaign money—the money that the Health Initiative could spend in the heat of the legislative session to lobby and run grassroots mobilization ads—chronically in short supply, for once was not. Late in the fall of 2003, DeMarco heard from Ellen Golmobek, the head of Americans for Health Care, an organization created by the politically aggressive Service Employees International Union (SEIU) then campaigning to expand health-care coverage in seven states. "We got on the radar screen of SEIU," DeMarco says. "I think all the publicity we were getting helped. They came to me, and I talked to them a long time; I described our plan. They liked it. They wanted to make it a priority. So they decided to give us a good amount of (c)(4) money, to supplement the other (c)(4) money we had. This would mean tens of thousands of dollars over the next few months. And the goal was to pass substantial health-care legislation in 2004."

DeMarco told the *Baltimore Sun*'s Salganik he was "thrilled" at the outlook: "We're going to have significant progress this year on health care." He was *almost* right. The legislation marched through the House and was actually strengthened by the Senate Finance Committee through the leadership of its chair, Senator Mac Middleton. The Senate bill needed twenty-four votes to pass. In 2003, twenty-nine senators had voted for a similar HMO tax.

Miller, the Spoiler Again—and Then the Hero

Victory seemed certain. But it wasn't. The failure of the House and Senate leadership to agree on the Busch-led House bill triggered the competitive resentment of Senate President Mike Miller to the House speaker's ascendancy, as well as Miller's fiscal conservatism. So as the legislative session was ending, Miller sabotaged yet another seemingly unstoppable DeMarco juggernaut. Miller had called in political obligations from senators who had benefited from his patronage, including five members of the Senate Budget and Taxation Committee who DeMarco and Schneider were sure stood with them. Schneider recalls the shock and misery at this outcome: "I remember Vinny just shaking his head, walking down out of the State House, just walking to our cars, and we didn't really say much. It was just like, Wow, what just happened?"

DeMarco brooded on the consequences of the bill's failure: "I just saw all these people's hard work gone down the tubes. It was gut-wrenching to come that close. Seventy thousand people—Glenn and I had done the numbers over again and thought how many people it would help. And I just kept thinking about the stories of people who don't have health care having their lives ruined, dying early, or going bankrupt. We could have done something. We were that close. It was very rough."

This time, however, he was not tempted to quit. Yet he had learned again the hard lesson that, no matter how fervent, the support of only one of the three most powerful inside leaders—the House speaker—was not enough in the face of resistance by the other two, the governor and the Senate president. Where to go next? As DeMarco ruminated over the wreckage of the 2004 session, one insight stuck with him: by itself, the proposed 8 percent payroll tax for employee health benefits on businesses with more than ten thousand employees had enjoyed strong support from the House and Senate committee leaders. Each had independently lifted it from the Health Initiative's comprehensive bill and added it to their own bills. But each chose not to include other provisions more onerous to smaller businesses.

DeMarco now recalled that "right in the beginning of the 2004 session, Senator Mac Middleton, chair of the Finance Committee, says, 'You know, there's a part of your plan I really like, the big-employer part.' That was my first indication that the big-employer tax was going to go off on its own." One of DeMarco's leaders, House committee chair Hurson, had become increasingly concerned with the finding in the economic report by the Lewin Group that the small-business requirement in the Health Initiative's full proposal would cause some job loss but would be offset by jobs gained in the health care sector. Lewin had also found that the 8 percent tax on the largest employers wouldn't lose *any* jobs, which was why Hurson included only that provision in this 2004 bill. What Glenn Schneider remembers about the evolution of Hurson's 2004 legislation was that "a peculiar thing was happening: this was the big bill of Hurson's career—to do this huge health-care expansion. So he held weekly work sessions, where he would go down different provisions and ask people what they thought. At one point, he asked the lobbyist for the retailers, 'How do you feel about this 8 percent payroll tax provision for the big employers?' And he said, 'We really don't have much of a problem with this part of the bill because it doesn't affect many of our retailers.'" The Health Initiative team was "pretty startled. We looked at each other as if to say, 'Did he just say that?' Then we realized that these folks were recognizing that this didn't affect too many businesses."

Now, as the 2005 session approached and DeMarco again consulted with key allies, he discovered that his labor allies were "thrilled" at the prospect of a law limited to the big employers, particularly the SEIU and the United Food and Commercial Workers (UFCW), whose large organized employers, especially Giant Food and Safeway, were being progressively undersold by nonunionized—and union-busting—Wal-Mart. One of the reasons Wal-Mart could undersell these stores was that it was not paying its "fair share" of employee health benefits. As a result, new allies like Giant Food and several small-business owners broadened visibly the active support for the bill.

The words "fair share" were especially apt in Maryland because of its unique "all-payer" hospital system, under which companies that paid adequate employee health insurance were required to pay part of their health insurance premiums to cover the hospitalization of the state's uninsured. These businesses were in effect subsidizing the health care of Wal-Mart's workforce, for Wal-Mart provided little health care for its large segment of temporary and part-time employees and insurance benefits so low to its regular employees, or premiums so high, that many were forced to seek public assistance. DeMarco's colleagues had calculated that this subsidy amounted to between 2 and 8 percent of the premiums the more responsible employers paid. Apart from Wal-Mart, the only business organizations in Maryland with more than ten thousand employees were Giant Food, Safeway, Johns Hopkins, and defense contractor Northrup Grumman, and each of these provided full health-care benefits for their employees.

The launching pad for DeMarco and Schneider's postmortem planning for the 2005 session was a new poll, funded by the SEIU. The Health Initiative released the results on January 12, 2005, just before the new legislative session opened: 78 percent of Maryland voters favored a law requiring companies with ten thousand or more employees to spend at least 8 percent of their payroll costs on health-care coverage. DeMarco was certain that a bill focused solely on this "fair share" concept could engage strong coalition support, especially among his labor allies. It could gain key business support from Wal-Mart competitor Giant Food and little or no opposition from unaffected smaller businesses. As for public support, the poll showed that the concept of "fairness" resonated strongly with voters. From that evidence, it was a short leap to frame and name the bill the "Fair Share bill," though the press would seize upon it as the "Wal-Mart bill."

Although it now made political good sense for the Health Initiative to focus squarely on the Fair Share bill for the 8 percent tax on the big companies and leave the Health Care for All! comprehensive bill for the day when a supportive governor took office, tension again arose within the coalition about setting aside the overall bill, Schneider says. "At every meeting, everyone said, 'We are in this because we believe in health care for all. Don't abandon that. Push the whole bill.'" But leading into the 2005 session, *all* agreed that it would also be worthwhile to put the big-company bill in, especially because of Giant's support. They could introduce and hold hearings on both bills, with a good chance of passing the narrow bill in either 2005 or 2006 while Ehrlich was still governor. Meanwhile, they could continue public education on the comprehensive bill, building longer-term support.

As the 2005 legislative session opened, the coalition members were motivated and mobilized, this time joined by an array of union lobbyists, as well as lobbyists for Giant Food. The UFCW's Mark Federici and Giant's Barry Scher walked the halls of Annapolis, ideologically arm-in-arm with DeMarco, buttonholing legislators to support the Fair Share bill. Perhaps best of all, as DeMarco says, "Mike Miller fell in love with Fair Share Health Care. He was our big ally. House Speaker Busch, too. Everybody. But it didn't happen right away."

> We did very intensive work throughout the 2005 session. We had sixty cosponsors in the House, many in the Senate. As the days went by in the session, we started to realize, this is a really hot thing. The public really likes it. In my lobbying, I kept hammering home as much as possible that businesses support the bill.
>
> Then we did the groundwork of identifying who the swing people were on the committees. And we pressed our coalition members to lobby them hard. It was grueling work for a month, two months. We finally got a great vote in the House committee; it kind of zoomed through the House floor. Then we knew the real battle was going to be on the Senate floor.
>
> There was a long, long debate on the Senate floor. Conservatives argued, "This is the first step toward socialized medicine." We fought off all amendments, including one potentially "killer" amendment that was spotted and blocked at the last minute by Senator Verna Jones, who later would become the lead Senate sponsor of our Health Care for All! legislation. Then it passed, thirty to seventeen.

The Perils of Flexibility

In fact, they did not fight off "all amendments." In his eagerness to win, DeMarco almost took flexibility a step too far to clear a nagging road-block to the passage of the Fair Share bill. Five employers in the state were large enough to be affected by the bill, but four of them paid health-care benefits that should have met the bill's standards; only Wal-Mart would be forced to double its health-care payments or pay an equivalent health-care assessment to the state. But the giant military aircraft manufacturer, Northrup Grumman, despite providing excellent health benefits that met the bill's intent, could well have been forced to pay more because its average salaries were uniquely high. Northrup Grumman demanded an exemption from the bill by amendment.

"I was open to that," DeMarco says, because if the bill got strong opposition from the highly influential Northrop Grumman, "we'd be dead."

But Glenn and everybody else said, "No way!" The policy wonks in the office and at SEIU said, "We don't want to screw up the whole Health Care for All! bill because of Fair Share." Glenn's point was, what happens when we work with companies under ten thousand? If we exclude the big companies now, we're going to have to exclude small companies down the road. If you exempt NG [Northrup Grumman], then you have to exempt Giant, et cetera. Then it truly would have been a Wal-Mart bill. People say it's only four companies, but in the future, we may have more companies that fit the bill.

DeMarco agonized but finally agreed: "Sometimes I do want to compromise too quickly, but how do we get the bill passed without sacrificing the principle? Not only for the future in Maryland, but the whole country's looking at this. I thought we were going to run into a train wreck. Because we couldn't agree on the NG amendment, NG was going to put its foot down in the Senate, which would kill us."

Then, an uncluttered mind stepped in. DeMarco's fourteen-year-old son, Tony, had a day off from school. "I took him with me to a hearing, and he heard debate on another bill. They were talking about median income, and I was talking about my conundrum, and he came up with an ingenious compromise." Tony's idea was to lower the threshold below which the 8 percent payroll tax would be applied from the Social Security tax threshold (about $100,000) to the state median income (about $55,000 at the time). This compromise would keep more of Northrup Grumman's high salaries from being assessed.

"We developed what I call the Tony DeMarco Amendment," DeMarco says. "It was introduced on the Senate floor by Senator DeGrange, because NG is in his district. (He hates my guts from the tobacco days.) He ended up voting against the bill, but we let him put in the amendment. And NG didn't raise a peep. They officially opposed the bill based on general principle, but they didn't go around slamming us. What would we have done if Tony hadn't saved my neck? I don't know. But that put us over the top."

In tallying the wins and losses of the 2005 session, the press widely acknowledged DeMarco's good year. Smith wrote a column in the April 24, 2005, *Sun* under the headline, "The Year of Vinnie, the Can't-Lose Lobbyist." Of the role of this "lobbyist extraordinaire" in the passage of this gaggle of healthcare bills, Smith wrote: "Many others were involved in these initiatives. But Mr. DeMarco and his Fair Share Health Care team were a constant." On April 17, 2005, Matthew Mosk and John Wagner of the *Washington Post* echoed Smith and added the prediction of a veto override: "Public interest lobbyist Vincent DeMarco has discovered the secret formula for getting tough bills through the legislature without any powerful backers. In past years, DeMarco muscled through a controversial trigger lock bill and a tobacco tax. This year, the rumpled lobbyist stuck it to Wal-Mart with a bill that would essentially force the retailer to increase health coverage for its workers. Ehrlich has pledged a veto, but with DeMarco involved, who would discount a possible override?"

DeMarco was too experienced in the dynamics of politics to forget that success would also require a measure of very good luck. That luck now came in the failed leadership of the chief adversary of the Fair Share bill, Governor Ehrlich. As Smith noted in his "Year of Vinnie" column, Ehrlich's unpopular political embrace of Wal-Mart and his equally unpopular threat of a veto were gifts to DeMarco: "Democrats rushed to pass the bill because they believed a veto would spotlight the governor as a friend of big corporate interests and an enemy of the little guy.... It adds up to a lobbyist's dream. The General Assembly's Democratic majority is often on Mr. DeMarco's side, and the Republican governor is on Mr. DeMarco's side whether he signs the bill or not."

The override vote would come in the first days of the 2006 legislative session. The week before, on January 6, Andrew Green noted in the *Baltimore Sun*: "Debate on the so-called Fair Share Health Care Act has drowned out nearly every other issue on the eve of this year's General Assembly session. National interest groups have poured money into the state, which is seen as a testing ground for whether similar legislation targeting the giant retailer [Wal-Mart] will succeed across the country." But Wal-Mart's lobbying fell short. Green wrote: "Jean B. Cryor of Montgomery County, the only Republican in either chamber to vote for the bill, said she had never heard from so many people on a bill before. But nothing she has heard has swayed her. 'If, indeed, I vote for a bill once, I would have to have something extraordinary happen to change my mind.'" Labor was broadly mobilized, and not just the affected unions. "The state AFL-CIO, led by their state president Fred Mason, did what they have never done before," DeMarco says. "They sent a letter to legislators saying, 'If you don't vote for this override, don't even bother asking for an endorsement. We won't even look at you.' This was astounding and I think that switched a couple of people. For a lot of these legislators, labor endorsement is a big thing."

So was business support. In addition to Giant's high-profile endorsement, there were op-ed columns in the *Baltimore Sun* and the *Washington Post* featuring prominent Baltimore developer Bill Struever, a moving-company owner named Mark Derbyshire from the conservative northern Baltimore suburbs, an auto shop owner named Brian England, and the owner of one of the oldest hardware stores in rural western Maryland, Jan Naylor—all recruited by DeMarco. Impressed by the effect of this support, DeMarco would make certain to greatly expand his outreach to business owners in future health-care reform efforts.

On January 12, 2006, both houses of the legislature voted to override the veto. In the House, the vote was eighty-eight to fifty, three more than needed. In the Senate, all fourteen Republicans voted with the governor, but thirty Democrats held firm, one more than needed. The next day, the *Sun*'s Green quoted DeMarco: "'Fair Share Health Care is going to sweep the nation,' said Vinny DeMarco. . . . 'This pro-business, pro-working families law makes sense, and the Maryland state legislature is taking the lead.'" National media—even international media—picked up the story as a new and promising approach to health-care expansion. DeMarco was quoted, in all his customary enthusiasm, in the *New York Times* and was featured on CNN and PBS's *NewsHour*. It was, DeMarco says, "the biggest thing I'd ever been involved in."

In April, Wal-Mart announced that it would cut in half the period that part-time employees had to wait to be eligible for health insurance. Wal-Mart also made the children of part-time employees eligible for health care and announced that copayments for some widely used prescription drugs would be reduced by 70 percent. "When our enrollment period opens this fall, many associates will see even lower premiums available than what they're paying today," a Wal-Mart representative told the *Sun*'s Andrew Green.

Six months after the veto override, a legal cloud rained on DeMarco's parade. On July 21, 2006, the U.S. District Court for the District of Maryland struck down the Fair Share law as violating the Federal Employee Retirement Income Security Act (ERISA), which governs employee benefit requirements. That law, the court held, preempts individual state efforts to regulate employee health benefits, including such legislation as the Fair Share law.

The bright side for DeMarco was his belief that the passage of the Fair Share law—and the threat that passage of such laws would cascade nationwide—had motivated Wal-Mart to make health-care improvements; as he told me, "It's not because of the legal impact around the law but because of the debate around the law that Wal-Mart found it necessary to expand health care."

Did DeMarco win a major victory with the passage of the Fair Share bill? Yes. Was the victory erased by the federal court? Yes. Did the success of the campaign continue to reverberate within Maryland and beyond to invigorate long-term momentum for the expansion of health care? Yes. Had Wal-Mart significantly improved its health-care benefits for its workers (though it was hardly yet a paragon of responsibility)? Yes. The key for DeMarco had been to follow his leaders within the legislature, even his chronic adversary, Senate President Miller—this time, in partnership with House Speaker Busch. Thus, the two legislative leaders rolled over the one leader whose support DeMarco would never have, Governor Ehrlich. DeMarco and the Maryland Health Care for All! Coalition had come back from the near dead.

In late July 2009, Barry Scher, now retired vice president of public affairs for Giant Food, wrote me:

> In 2006, while I was the chief lobbyist for the largest food chain in Maryland, we agreed to help Vinny DeMarco fight to make all Maryland businesses pay their fair share for the health care of their employees, which Wal-Mart refused to do. Vinny was relentless in his pursuit because he said what he believed in and even though Wal-Mart hired the biggest guns to lobby on their behalf, even they could not quell the fight. So when the *Wall Street Journal* of July 1, 2009, appeared on the street, with the headline, "Wal-Mart Backs Drive to Make Companies Pay for Health Coverage," it made me think of the power of Vinny. Never in my wildest dreams did I think Wal-Mart would change their position so drastically. And to think it all started in Maryland with Vinny DeMarco as the leader for health care reform.

9

Coming to Terms
with a Governing Troika

Long before the 2006 Maryland General Assembly overrode the governor's veto of the Fair Share law, even before the 2005 General Assembly passed the Fair Share bill itself, DeMarco was planning his next campaign: "One of the things I've learned over the years is that it's important to think about your next steps—to have it started in your head—while you're still doing the step you're in, not waiting until you're done." DeMarco began to focus, once again, on raising the cigarette tax, this time to expand Medicaid coverage for the low-income parents of children covered under the State Children's Health Insurance Program. But he felt that the thirty-six-cent increase in the cigarette tax already contained in the Health Care for All! comprehensive plan was not substantial enough as a smoking prevention measure—nor large enough to fund health-care expansion significant enough to engage and energize the coalition. The early polling that the Campaign for Tobacco-Free Kids had funded had shown that voter support didn't change whether the increase was thirty-six cents, a dollar, or even two dollars. DeMarco consulted with his key coalition allies and Hopkins health-care experts and then settled upon a one-dollar increase, to be dedicated to expanding Medicaid coverage.

Why not a general tax increase to fund Medicaid expansion? Two reasons, says DeMarco. First, general tax increases are unpopular. Second, everybody wants part of the proceeds, which could pit Health Care for All! against advocacy groups for education, transportation, and so on. "I'd rather be fighting [tobacco lobbyist] Bruce Bereano than the Maryland State Teachers Association any day," DeMarco says.

DeMarco knew that he would again need the active support of strong legislative leaders, even if, as he hoped, Governor Ehrlich did not win reelection. In any event, in 2005 and 2006, he would still face Ehrlich, a governor completely opposed to both a cigarette tax increase and Medicaid expansion. He would still face a Senate president hostile to cigarette tax increases and wary of health-care expansion in a time of budget crunch. As DeMarco says, "It had to be Mike Busch," the House speaker and the only other strong leader. Yet despite Busch's commitment to health-care expansion—"the whole Fair Share battle really helped make him a friend and ally"—Busch had reservations about the fairness of cigarette tax increases.

"Leery" is how DeMarco describes Busch in their first meetings on the cigarette tax/Medicaid proposal: Busch was convinced that cigarette taxes penalize lower-income people who were still smoking. "You're hurting the people who are already addicted," he told DeMarco. His were among "the most sincere concerns about the tobacco tax I've ever heard from a public official," DeMarco says. Promising to supply Busch with information that raising the cost of smoking helps the poor rather than hurts them, DeMarco set out to "bring Mike Busch along."

He had one "inside" ally, Kristin Jones, a Busch staff assistant and a quiet supporter of the cigarette tax/Medicaid concept. Even more, DeMarco needed the support of the House colleague whom the speaker most trusted on matters of health, Peter Hammen. Busch had picked Hammen to chair the House Health and Government Operations Committee "for a reason," says DeMarco. "Busch *liked* him." When DeMarco talked to Hammen, Hammen immediately said he had no problem with the tobacco tax but he wondered whether Medicaid expansion would fund drug treatment, a deep concern for him. "A woman in South Baltimore had told him that her son's life was being destroyed," DeMarco says, because "he couldn't get treatment." Their answer was: "Fund Medicaid as well as drug treatment. Look, Medicaid covers drug treatment, though not as fully as other drug programs. But when you put a dollar into Medicaid, you get a dollar match from the federal government. That's two dollars for drug treatment as well as other health coverage."

DeMarco, Schneider, and Lucchi spent time reaching out to Mike Busch and Pete Hammen in 2005. "Mike Busch hadn't been sold yet, but he appreciated us talking with him, and he said he'd think about it," says DeMarco. "We knew that if Pete Hammen was for it that would bring Mike Busch a long way. The two of them talk all the time." Nothing DeMarco would do in this campaign would be more important than this effort to enlist Busch not just as a supporter, but as a champion of the tax increase/Medicaid expansion.

Hammen and many others the DeMarco team was talking to warned against expanding Medicaid without recognizing the budget gap that the Medicaid program already faced in Maryland. DeMarco opted for what he calls a "fiscally conservative" proposal, which became the basis for an organizing resolution for the one-dollar tax increase. This would raise about $200 million, put tens of millions into filling the budget hole in Medicaid, and then fund a major expansion of Medicaid to cover the parents of children involved in the State Children's Health Insurance Program—to guarantee a federal match. "We didn't even think about doing non-parents," says DeMarco, "because it was too much money." The benefits they proposed went beyond Medicaid, though, to broaden support with money earmarked for drug treatment, tobacco control, grants to small businesses to help them provide health care, and health disparities.

To those in the Health Care for All! Coalition who complained that now the goal had shrunk to a tobacco tax for only fifty thousand to one hundred thousand people, leaving seven hundred thousand still uninsured, DeMarco answered: "Ehrlich's governor. What can we do? We've got to do what we can do." This new proposal was now newly baptized by DeMarco and his team as the Healthy Maryland Initiative.

The 2006 Elections

With the approach of the 2006 elections, the Healthy Maryland Initiative moved forward with the resolution, pledge signings, and the other signature stages from DeMarco's strategic template. The Democratic gubernatorial candidates challenging incumbent Bob Ehrlich—Martin O'Malley and Douglas Duncan—loomed large in the campaign's sights. Although DeMarco was not close to O'Malley, he admired his successes as mayor of Baltimore and welcomed his general support for health-care expansion. Duncan signed the tobacco tax/Medicaid expansion campaign pledge and O'Malley did not. The initiative heralded Duncan's support, but soon thereafter, Duncan's poor health caused him to drop out of the race. DeMarco now began to reach out to O'Malley as best he could, finding an opening first with O'Malley's chief communications staffer, Rick Abbruzzese. Although Abbruzzese was himself open to a tobacco tax increase, he told DeMarco that O'Malley was "not going to support it now." Abbruzzese agreed to keep talking about it with DeMarco after the election, and their growing relationship would prove helpful to both the new governor and the Healthy Maryland Initiative. Meanwhile, with Abbruzzese's help, DeMarco said, candidate O'Malley "was careful never to be too negative about the initiative but just to express concerns about health care being funded by a declining revenue source like a tobacco tax effort."

The health-care campaign now faced a situation it had never confronted before. "Even in 2002 before Kathleen [Kennedy Townsend] lost, we had a gubernatorial candidate who supported the proposal," DeMarco points out. "We didn't this time." Yes, they had House Health and Government Operations Committee chair Pete Hammen. They also had the reassurance of House

Speaker Mike Busch. "Busch told us," says DeMarco, "he was not signing any-thing, but he told us, 'You're going to get something.'" As DeMarco read it, Hammen would not have signed the pledge if Mike Busch had wanted him not to. "I think two things happened with Mike Busch," DeMarco says. "I think we met his concerns on the tobacco tax, and I think he started to understand how this would be a great way to expand health care." What Speaker Busch doubtless also understood—and appreciated—was that the 2006 elections had accelerated the momentum for health-care expansion. Almost everything in DeMarco's plan, including his furious campaigning, was in place for ac-tion. Democrats had kept 33 of the 47 Senate seats. Democrats gained 6 House seats, bringing their majority to 104 of the 141 members. Martin O'Malley would be the new governor.

"The Bill Passed—Just Not Yet"

As the legislature convened in January 2007, roughly half of both houses—seventy-eight votes—were already committed to the Healthy Mary-land Initiative's plan. House Speaker Busch, with Health and Government Operations Committee chair Hammen, seized the legislative leadership to advocate the cigarette tax/Medicaid legislation. They had privately let it be known, says Glenn Schneider, that "they don't necessarily want to be seen as being pushed around by this Health Care for All! Coalition, but they certainly want to work closely with us." The House leaders held a press conference to announce that they were introducing a bill of their own, even broader than the comprehensive Healthy Maryland bill but nonetheless embracing the cigarette tax and other elements of the Initiative's plan.

As the session got under way, DeMarco arranged for the Healthy Mary-land Initiative to recognize Hammen's leadership at a Martin Luther King Day event. "Matt [Celentano] and Glenn constantly harass me for giving awards before people do what we need them to do," DeMarco said, "but I look at an award as an incentive. And I thought Pete was the right person to give this award to." Later, Hammen told DeMarco that the tobacco tax would "definitely be in the House bill" and that he would push it in his own plan. Hammen advised him, DeMarco says, "'Don't worry about the House; spend all your lobbying on the Senate.'"

That was good advice. There remained two massive roadblocks to enact-ment of the Healthy Maryland Initiative's bill in the 2007 regular session: the governor and the Senate president. The new governor, O'Malley, had sup-ported health-care expansion, but in his first legislative proposal as governor, he came up with a very limited health-care proposal—with no cigarette tax and no Medicaid expansion.

Senate President Miller continued to oppose cigarette tax increases, as he had in 1999. But there were competing pressures on him in 2007, including the huge budget deficit that loomed on the state's horizon; Miller began to eye health-care expansion as a potential popular political sweetener for a near certain broad tax increase to pay for closing the gap. Miller also hung on to the dream he had advocated for many years, only to be frustrated by House Speaker Busch: to legalize slot machines to produce a new tax windfall. Over several sessions, slots versus no slots had become a contest of wills between the two strong leaders.

DeMarco feared that Miller would stonewall the Initiative's cigarette tax and Medicaid plan, at least during the 2007 session—not because he unalterably opposed raising the cigarette tax, but because he was holding his support hostage to Busch's acquiescence to slots. So DeMarco at this point had only one of the three leaders in his corner—Busch, who was fully committed. The second, Miller, was firmly opposed, at least for this session; and the third, Governor O'Malley, was all but opposed—for now.

On February 17, 2007, ninety witnesses testified before Hammen's House Health and Government Operations Committee. Besides DeMarco, they included representatives from the Smoke Free Coalition, including Bonita Pennino of the American Cancer Society and Michaeline Fedder of the American Heart Association, other key partners such as Quincey Gamble of 1199 SEIU, Dr. Marty Wasserman of the Medical Society, and Joe DeMattos of the American Association of Retired Persons (AARP), along with faith and community leaders from across the state. In addition, the Maryland Hospital Association and the Greater Baltimore Committee (a politically influential business group) helped considerably by separately endorsing a one-dollar tobacco tax proposal to expand Medicaid. Of the ninety witnesses, only a handful—all cigar dealers—opposed the bill. Speaker Busch appeared at Hammen's hearing to support the bill—a rare presence for the speaker that signaled to all his deep commitment. After calling health-care expansion "a laudable goal that we ought to try to accomplish," he stayed to listen.

The key organizations did more than appear at the hearing. From the SEIU, a mailing went out to hundreds of thousands of people urging them to press legislators to support the tobacco tax for health care. AARP's members made their support felt all over Annapolis, including in Senate President Mike Miller's office. The premier national health-care organization, Families USA, helped out by funding an ad that focused on how the health-care expansion would reduce the "hidden health-care tax" that Marylanders all pay to cover the hospitalization of the uninsured. All this orchestrated advocacy was building pressure on the legislature, including its leaders.

As chair, Hammen now consolidated the various bills presented to the House Health and Government Operations Committee into a single consensus committee bill, with the Healthy Maryland Initiative's tax and other provisions intact. The Hammen bill expanded health care significantly beyond the initiative's bill by putting all the tobacco tax money into Medicaid expansion and none into building up Medicaid deficit reduction. DeMarco and most of his allies were thrilled, although some were upset that Hammen had not specifically allocated any of the Medicaid money for drug treatment, small businesses, tobacco control, or health disparities. In the end, DeMarco rallied the Health Care for All! Coalition behind the Hammen bill as the best way to expand health care in Maryland and maximize the federal matching money. The bill, as DeMarco says, came "roaring out of the House by a whopping 102 to 37 vote. Then the speaker does a big press conference. And then, of course, it goes to the Senate, and then we have that knocky-heads. We have a big press conference with faith leaders, demanding the Senate do this. We put on the pressure. But we kept hearing from senators, 'It's not going to happen this year.'"

The bill never emerged from the Senate committee. As the days of the session dwindled down, DeMarco e-mailed me: "I am feeling a combination of let down and exhilarated at the same time. Unlike the 1998 'trial run' situation, we really wanted to get it done this year, as did the House leadership, so it is hard not to feel somewhat down about it. But, it is clear that our coalition and electoral work have made health-care expansion right at the top of the agenda in Maryland and I am feeling very good about it happening next time."

Still, as the session ended, DeMarco went home more let down than exhilarated. His son Jamie comforted him. "Don't worry, Dad," he assured his father. "The bill passed—just not yet."

One Down, Two to Go

The failure of the cigarette tax/Medicaid expansion effort in the regular 2007 General Assembly session challenged DeMarco's belief that he didn't need the support of all three key legislative leaders to get what he wanted if one of them—the governor, the speaker of the House, or the president of the Senate—also *really* wanted it. Perhaps if the other two had cared less in this case, DeMarco might have been right. But while Speaker Busch now *really* wanted the cigarette tax increase to pay for the Medicaid expansion, Governor O'Malley and Senate President Miller *really* didn't. Hence, stalemate.

The rationale both O'Malley and Miller publicly expressed for opposing the coupling of a cigarette tax and Medicaid expansion was the anticipated decline in cigarette tax revenues as higher tobacco prices discouraged consumption. Miller's resistance also flowed from his resentment at DeMarco's relentless pushing, which erupted in his outburst during an interview for public radio: "Martin O'Malley should be making health-care policy in Maryland, not Vinny DeMarco." DeMarco would have to find a way to overcome the resistance of both the governor and the Senate president to the Initiative's proposal.

Shifting Tactics, Shifting Credit

Through conversations with Governor O'Malley's staff members, with whom DeMarco by now had developed a good working relationship, and through Healthy Maryland Initiative lobbyist Len Lucchi's soundings of Senate President Mike Miller's staff, DeMarco learned that both leaders were open to health-care expansion. O'Malley, indeed, was ready to call a Special Session in the fall to deal with the looming budget deficit crisis, with his own health-care expansion plan as the sweetener to offset the sour taste of higher taxes and budget cuts.

At this point, DeMarco realized that if the Initiative could *separately* achieve the Medicaid expansion it sought *and* the full one-dollar cigarette tax increase, that would be a major public health achievement—even if the two weren't tied together. His strategy in linking them had sprung all along from his belief that the legislature would never authorize the Medicaid expansion without the tax as a dedicated source of funding. Now it appeared possible, even likely, that he could achieve both by losing his battle to treat them as a unit. He could win by losing—by allowing O'Malley and Miller to claim that the independent health and tax initiatives were theirs, not Vinny DeMarco's.

Now, ironically, DeMarco's greatest lobbying challenge would be not the governor and the Senate president, but his own coalition. Over the summer of 2007, he had to convince his allies that the link they had fought for between the cigarette tax and Medicaid expansion was no longer necessary. The Healthy Maryland Initiative would remain publicly committed to the link but would encourage and welcome O'Malley's proposals. Some key initiative leaders objected to unlinking the tobacco tax and health-care expansion, both because they wanted to prevent Miller from tying health-care expansion to slot machines and because they felt that tobacco tax increases were the only secure way to fund such expansion. DeMarco finally persuaded them that getting and keeping the support of Miller and O'Malley depended on separating the two.

Confirmation that this was a sound strategic direction began to come in. In an August 12 article, the *Sun*'s Andrew Green quoted O'Malley. "You have to be very, very poor indeed to be on Medicaid in this state," the governor said, and he announced his intention to seek expanded Medicaid coverage. Later in the piece, headlined "O'Malley Favors Medicaid Growth," DeMarco, bypassing the funding question, was quoted hailing the governor as the savior of health-care reform: "It's great news for the people of Maryland. Thousands of Marylanders can't get the health care they need, and everyone pays through the hospitalization of the uninsured." He did not comment on O'Malley's expressed doubts about the merit of a tobacco tax increase.

Nevertheless, as DeMarco had expected, in Governor O'Malley's search for politically attainable sources of funding to meet the budget shortfall, he eventually seized the popular high ground. On September 8, O'Malley said in a radio interview: "I do think there is the will to raise the tobacco tax. We will probably see some sort of increase." DeMarco's strategy was now fixed; he agreed with the governor: "We commend Governor O'Malley for expressing support for the one-dollar tobacco tax increase. By itself, it will keep fifty thousand kids from smoking, save thousands of lives from tobacco-caused deaths, and save the state billions of dollars in health-care costs."

One to Go: Swallowing Slots

O'Malley also met Senate President Miller halfway. He acknowledged slot machines "as a necessary component of the budget solution," Green also reported in his August 12 *Sun* article. House Speaker Busch reiterated his aversion to slots, Green reported, but "expects members of his chamber would be more flexible in supporting new revenue measures if they are tied to health care expansion, environmental protections and other measures to improve the quality of life in Maryland."

"We're hoping the stars are aligned," DeMarco told the *Washington Post*'s Lisa Rein by September 12. With the Special Session set to open on October 30, he had both Speaker Busch and Governor O'Malley leading his fight. That left Senate President Miller, whose support still hinged on slots. Though DeMarco had never campaigned against slot machines, like Busch he personally opposed them as an invisible regressive tax on low-income workers. Yet DeMarco, as well as O'Malley and Busch, understood that Miller would insist on slots as a precondition to his agreeing to any health-care expansion. Busch came up with the compromise that broke the logjam—putting the slots issue before the voters through a statewide referendum. Governor O'Malley quickly agreed to this, and Miller reluctantly went along. Though he continued to dislike slots, DeMarco determined that his health coalition had to stay out of this fight. Faith leaders would fight even the proposal to put slots on the ballot, but others in the coalition, including the AFL-CIO, strongly supported allowing slot machines in Maryland. DeMarco resisted all efforts to get the Healthy Maryland Initiative involved—though his holding out proved painful.

Most troubling to DeMarco was the concern expressed by many in the faith community, including his strong allies the United Methodists, that the health-care expansion would be tied to slots. DeMarco made clear the coalition's position of what he called "aggressive neutrality" on the slots issue. "As I discussed," DeMarco wrote to one United Methodist leader, "there was an attempt to make the health care bill contingent on the passage of the slots referendum. We strongly opposed that and it was not done. Partly because of our strong opposition, the governor's health care bill does not link any health care expansion to slots."

But the compromise leading to a state referendum on slots was still troubling. Discontent within the Healthy Maryland campaign with DeMarco's and the coalition's neutrality would not disappear, despite DeMarco's delicate dance, but there would be no rebellion. Most important, Senate President Miller was finally satisfied. He, the governor, and the House speaker were at last joined in their determination to fight together for the governor's package—including cigarette taxes and Medicaid expansion. DeMarco had his three leaders. Although some coalition partners cautioned DeMarco against praising the governor before they knew exactly what he was going to propose, Speaker Busch's aide Kristin Jones told DeMarco that his strategy of publicly supporting the governor was paving the way toward bringing everyone together around a strong health-care proposal.

More evidence that the momentum was now unstoppable came in this frustrated plaint from tobacco lobbyist Bruce Bereano, that ubiquitous DeMarco nemesis, to the Montgomery County *Gazette*'s Douglas Tallman on September 28: "On the tobacco tax, I'm really frustrated and disturbed there's this continuous attack on people that use tobacco and smoke," Bereano said. "All these Vinnie DeMarco crazies. They're anti-tobacco and that is their agenda and they feel, foolishly I believe, if you raise the price, you're going to stop people from smoking." But most remarkable of all was this tiny note buried in Tallman's "Reporter's Notebook," a parallel column, the same day: "Mike Miller called across State Circle to health lobbyist Vinnie DeMarco . . . as he was entering his car for a trip to his Prince George's County office, 'Vinnie, I'm trying to get health care for you!'"

On November 19, 2007, the Senate voted to commit $280 million to the expansion of the state's health-care system. The final vote: thirty in favor, fourteen opposed. After he had sent out a press release to all the media, DeMarco broadcast an e-mail message to "Healthy Maryland Initiative Supporters": "Now, we can build on this success to achieve our goal of quality, affordable health care for all Marylanders—but first, rest, have a great Thanksgiving and Holiday Season and CELEBRATE!"

How Significant?

What was the significance of the work of the Healthy Maryland Initiative and its allies? There would be much media notice of the health action taken during this Special Session. The Maryland correspondent of the conservative *Washington Times*, Tom LoBianco, in a piece on November 29, 2007, noted that the legislation put the state "at the forefront of national health care reform," according to "members of the Democrat-controlled General Assembly." He quoted House Speaker Mike Busch: "Health care coverage has been an issue that consistently comes back in all the polling that people want addressed. That's why states have taken it on themselves to come up with an answer to the uninsured problem."

DeMarco was not quite finished courting Governor O'Malley. On December 15, a large ad in the *Baltimore Sun* featured a smiling group portrait of the governor and General Assembly leadership. Headlined "Message from the Maryland Citizens Health Initiative Education 2007 Fund: Thank you, Governor O'Malley and the General Assembly!," it read: "Historic Expansion of Health Insurance to 100,000 Uninsured; Assistance for Small Businesses to Provide Health Insurance; Doubling of Tax on Cigarettes to Discourage Teen Smoking." The message concluded with a quotation from O'Malley's health secretary, John Colmers: "This is foundational work. Then we can further whittle away at the rest of the 750,000 uninsured."

Once More into the Breach

A week before the Special Session voted on the governor's package, when the fate of DeMarco's last two years of strenuous effort was out of his hands, he began to prepare for the next—perhaps final—campaign to achieve the long-term goal of health care for all Marylanders. The skeptical columnist Fraser Smith, who had watched and analyzed DeMarco's campaigns, through failure and success, for more than twenty years, had become a believer: "Given his track record, it is unlikely anyone will bet against him."

With each of his incremental gains in expanding health-care coverage, did DeMarco also achieve sustained momentum toward Peter Beilenson's initial goal of universal health care for all Marylanders? As this narrative ends, it's too early to tell. But on September 17, 2008, I received this e-mail message from Leonard Lucchi, who is not often given to exuberance. Lucchi had just watched DeMarco present to key administration and legislative leaders his 2009 health care for all plan, which built upon the recent Medicaid expansion success:

> What happened was extraordinary. Not only did the staff members attend the briefing yesterday, but so did the House and Senate Committee Chairmen with jurisdiction over health care, their key colleagues on their committees, the State Health Secretary, the Governor's health advisor, and key staff members for the Speaker and Senate President.
>
> Vinny had a panel of experts from Hopkins describe the plan. Except for some facial contortions when the list of new taxes was described, there were no outbursts. Vinny let the Hopkins guys explain the plan and only interjected for some occasional political spin. After the presentation, there was a pregnant pause. I fully expected Vinny to be led from the room in handcuffs or at least for the legislators to ask if he was crazy. Instead, the Senate Chairman said that the legislature has a "moral obligation" to provide health care to everyone and had a "moral obligation" to work on Vinny's plan. This Senator is a farmer who represents a rural area and is somewhat conservative. Then the House Chairman said that he believes there are pieces of the plan that can be adopted over the next two years until the time is right to adopt the whole thing. Then the State Health Secretary agreed that this was what needed to be done over time.
>
> Today, Vinny got a call from committee staff asking for information to begin drafting parts of his plan for a 2009 bill. With previous plans, Vinny couldn't even get in the room and when he did, he was cursed at. (I am exaggerating to make the point.) This time, no one even second-guessed whether this was the direction to go in. The difference is that the legislature, by adopting Vinny's health bill during the special session, is now committed to finding a way to reach the ultimate objective. It's like being a little bit pregnant—it is impossible. Amazingly, the debate as to whether the state should even seek the goal of universal health care is now over.

Part III

A Leap of Faith Organizing

In Parts I and II, I looked at DeMarco's roles as leader and principal strategist in policy campaigns. Now, I turn to his contribution in a secondary support role developing a broader advocacy movement. These two chapters chronicle the ways in which the DeMarco factor helped transform the state and the national tobacco control movement, most uniquely by building an alliance between traditional public health advocates and faith community advocates across the political spectrum.

Chapter 10 tells of the organization of a network of national faith leaders to engage in focused policy advocacy in support of central tobacco control health policy objectives. Chapter 11 illustrates how DeMarco and his colleagues at the national Campaign for Tobacco-Free Kids helped strengthen state tobacco control advocacy, in large part by drawing on this organized network of national leaders to facilitate the mobilizing of state networks of faith leaders to the cause. Finally, we witness the deployment of the national faith leadership and the empowered state faith and health alliances to put convincing nonpartisan political pressure on their congressional representatives to enact comprehensive FDA regulation of tobacco manufacturing and marketing.

10

The Birth of Faith
United Against Tobacco

From their first meeting, Vincent DeMarco "loved" Peter Fisher of the national Campaign for Tobacco-Free Kids (TFK), whose job was to assist states in their tax increase and other campaigns. Engrossed at the time with the MCI campaign, DeMarco also began to consult with Carter Headrick ("Great guy!"), TFK's mid-Atlantic coordinator charged with helping state coalitions with their campaigns. He credits Fisher and Headrick, along with Glenn Schneider, with teaching him "everything I needed to know" about the tobacco issue. They helped him through the MCI campaign with grant money, DeMarco says, "and a lot of good advice."

By 1999, DeMarco began to return the favor, bringing advocacy strategies he had honed in Maryland to the aid of TFK's efforts in other states. TFK was staffed with veteran tobacco control advocates, joined by experienced advocates from other fields such as media advocacy. It was well funded by The Robert Wood Johnson Foundation and the American Cancer Society—at $12 million a year, enough to go toe-to-toe with the tobacco lobbyists, if not with tobacco's massive advertising budgets. Its mission was to serve both as a more potent Washington tobacco control lobby and as a resource to state tobacco control coalitions.

The election of George W. Bush in 2000, along with tobacco-friendly Republican control of both the Senate and the House, came as a blow to TFK's plan to pursue significant federal tobacco control legislation. Because many state-level efforts were not similarly afflicted, TFK's leaders decided to expand to promising state endeavors the kind of successful support they had provided Maryland and to broaden the nature of that support.

Fisher called DeMarco early in 2001. Would he be willing to serve as a consultant on the TFK team to work with tobacco control advocates in a couple of promising but stalled states? The goal was to help generate campaigns modeled on MCI. DeMarco agreed. He started with a handful of states chosen by Fisher and the TFK regional field team—community organizers working with state tobacco control advocates around the country. As in Maryland, DeMarco began by reaching out and developing a close working relationship with his new colleagues—Fisher and each field team member he would be working with. He learned whom among TFK's expert staff he could turn to for technical support, ranging from video press releases to solid, research-based, well-framed answers to virtually any tobacco control challenge. And he began reaching out to key state tobacco control leaders whom his TFK colleagues identified as effective partners.

Even with strong support, DeMarco soon reached the limits of his nearly boundless energy as he tried to clone his hands-on, state-organizing modus operandi in one new state after another, simultaneously juggling a flock of fledgling campaigns. He also encountered new obstacles. Unlike the scenario in Maryland, where the desperate Smoke Free Maryland Coalition had been ready to embrace new and more aggressive electoral strategies, advocates in these states, as in most, were wary of the electoral process engagement central to DeMarco's strategy. Most of their funding came from tax-exempt philanthropic sources or state governments, sources excessively skittish about funding political activity. They were more enthusiastic about DeMarco's ideas for broadening their coalitions, including outreach to the faith community. But, DeMarco laments, the advocates never seemed to build the desire to reach out on their own.

He soon realized he didn't have time to do enough outreach in all the states himself, yet he clung to his initial determination: "From the beginning, from day one, I said to Pete, 'Look, we've got to get the faith community involved as part of a broader movement.'" By now, he had sensed among the faith groups he had approached in various states the same enthusiasm he had earlier found in the faith community in Maryland. He realized that he could "get some of the national faith leaders connected with their state people, and then use that connection to build state faith and tobacco coalitions." He had worked with the national leadership on the gun issue, especially the United Methodists. When he was at Handgun Control, Inc., he had built a national coalition to oppose repeal of the assault weapons ban and "got most of the national groups, including the Catholics, aboard." So just as at the state level in Maryland, he had a ready-made connection with national faith groups.

He convinced Pete Fisher that they should meet with Jim Winkler, the relatively new general secretary of the United Methodist's General Board of Church and Society—one of the highest-ranking laypeople in the church hierarchy. They invited Patricia Sosa, TFK's vice president for outreach and grassroots organizing, to join them for what turned out to be, DeMarco says, a "great meeting." It led to a strategy session convened by Winkler with other senior leaders of the national United Methodist Church, who all expressed keen interest in helping TFK make tobacco control a top priority for all faith communities and, in particular, helping replicate in key states the "Maryland model" of faith mobilizing. Winkler would prove to be the ideal ally and leader. He was a seasoned advocate, knew the informal network of faith leaders well, and was highly respected by them. He welcomed the opportunity to join forces with TFK to help mobilize and focus the political energy of faith groups, which took so many positions on public policy issues that focus was a chronic problem.

For DeMarco, as propitious as the meeting with Winkler was connecting with Patricia Sosa, who told him that TFK had reached out to the faith community in the past but had never really tried mobilizing their ranks. From the very beginning of her work with DeMarco, Sosa says, theirs "was a bridge-building project between public health and faith." Together they developed a plan, with Winkler and other faith leaders they knew, to build a network of national faith leaders and persuade them, says DeMarco, to muster their members nationwide around raising cigarette taxes and all other tobacco control initiatives. Along with Sosa, DeMarco would be as relentless and resourceful in building this alliance as he had proved to be in building each of his coalitions in Maryland. Drawing from his Maryland template, the two crafted a resolution that would have broad ecumenical appeal: a pledge of support for raising tobacco taxes at the state level. In January 2002, together with Jim Winkler and other faith leaders, they formally launched Faith United Against Tobacco.

DeMarco and Sosa wrote letters; convened meetings to plan other meetings and events; held breakfasts, lunches, and press conferences; spoke and recruited at the meetings and conferences of other organizations—all culminating in a lengthening list of signatories to the resolution. Eventually, they would recruit more than two dozen national faith denominations and organizations as active members of Faith United Against Tobacco, including Christian, Jewish, Muslim, Sikh, and interdenominational groups such as the National Council of Churches and the National Association of Evangelicals. Theologically, and politically, they broadly encompassed both liberal and conservative.

The Ones That Almost Got Away

Although DeMarco and Sosa did not believe they had to recruit *every* faith group in the country, there were two church hierarchies outside the traditional mainstream National Council of Churches that they sorely needed—

the Catholic and the Southern Baptist. These were among the most politically potent outliers from the mainstream, mostly liberal churches. "We knew we had to break that barrier," DeMarco explains. "At least one of the two."

The Catholics

"When we speak with other tobacco control advocates, especially when we go to regional tobacco control meetings or the national meeting and we talk about faith outreach," Sosa says, "the advocates always ask, 'Where is the Catholic Church?'" The largest denomination in the country, the Catholics are well organized, she says, and less divided than the more numerous Protestants. The highly bureaucratic structure of the Catholic Church is a plus, she has found. "Once you get hold of the leadership of the Church, you really can do a lot. The way you do it is you actually go to the U.S. Conference of Catholic Bishops," the governing body of the Catholic Church in the United States.

DeMarco and Sosa tried just that—not once, but on several occasions. But they ran into a stone wall with policy staff, who insisted that the conference focused only on grand social issues like poverty and social justice. The Church runs a huge hospital system and has been a strong presence on health policy issues, but, says Sosa, she and DeMarco were never "able to break through and get them to even consider a policy on tobacco." Then they learned of another avenue to Catholic public policy leadership. More than thirty states have their own Catholic conference, with a lay executive director who is at the center of lobbying activity in that state. These executive directors had developed their own policy networks, and twice each year they gathered in Washington to interact on federal and state issues.

How DeMarco proceeded to work around the Conference of Catholic Bishops, Sosa recounts, was "*so* Vinny!" His interstate networking had brought him in touch with the Maine tobacco control coalition, one of the most successful in the country. Through that group he had met and befriended the Catholic lobbyist in Maine, Marc Mutty, who had been a vigorous activist in the Maine coalition. DeMarco asked Mutty to help identify Catholic lobbyists in other states also committed to tobacco control, and then he asked whether Mutty would be willing to call these colleagues to open the door to the other state executive directors for DeMarco and Sosa. He did that—and more.

DeMarco also had a relationship with the executive director of the Maryland Catholic Conference, Dick Dowling, from his Maryland gun control campaign days. Though tobacco was not a high priority for this director, he was willing to help DeMarco connect with other state directors who might be potential allies. Their networking, with critical help from TFK's Amy Barkley, eventually put DeMarco and Sosa in touch with the Kentucky Catholic Conference executive director, Ed Monahan, who quickly became, Sosa says, "a real role model for the other Catholic executive directors." Because Monahan comes from a tobacco state, he could rebut the concern of those in the Catholic Conference that members in tobacco states would be offended by tobacco control advocacy. Monahan "makes a very compelling case in terms of the links between tobacco consumption, smoking rates, and the burden of Medicaid and the growth of Medicaid expenditures," Sosa says. "He's bought into our entire agenda, from tax increases to federal regulation of the tobacco companies."

By December 2005, DeMarco had five Catholic Conference state executive directors—from Maine, Kentucky, Maryland, Illinois, and Indiana—fully engaged and feisty. He persuaded them to seek a meeting with the head of the policy shop for the Conference of Catholic Bishops to plead for elevating tobacco control as a national priority, and the directors in turn invited DeMarco and Sosa to join them. Sosa reports that the policy head said she didn't think it was the right time to bring the issue to the conference but added: "Let me tell you what I'm willing to do. If anybody reaches out to me and says tobacco is an issue we should cover, I would definitely encourage them to do it. I will."

As Sosa says, this was progress: "She was not saying no. She was saying, 'Yes, we will encourage the state directors to do it.'" The five state directors already onboard agreed to recruit their colleagues. Monahan from Kentucky and Mutty from Maine wrote letters that DeMarco took to other Catholic Conferences, such as Alaska's. The executive director there, Sosa says, is now working with TFK and the Alaska coalition.

The Southern Baptists (If at first . . .)

If the U.S. Conference of Catholic Bishops was, at first, a stone wall, the Southern Baptists were an impenetrable fortress. Rev. Cynthia Abrams, the Methodists' national tobacco control advocate, had built alliances with more conservative churches on such common-ground issues as pornography, gambling, and alcohol. So Abrams arranged for DeMarco and Sosa to meet with the Southern Baptists' chief Washington lobbyist and accompanied them to the meeting—a "complete disaster" that still makes DeMarco shudder. He was told that the Southern Baptists cared only about three issues besides judicial appointments, as DeMarco puts it: "stopping abortion, stopping gay marriage, stopping cloning." Other health issues? Oh, no, "abortion, cloning, and gay marriage, that's it." DeMarco says he knew that they were thinking, "These are not our kind of people." What DeMarco was thinking was, "Well, that's going to be tough."

Still, DeMarco and Sosa kept looking for an opening to the Southern Baptists. The United Methodist's Jim Winkler, who had become the chair of Faith United and a strong voice for outreach to unlikely allies, encouraged them not to lose hope. "I do recall saying at that point that we were very much at odds with the Southern Baptists over … the war in Iraq. Dr. Land [the spokesman for the Southern Baptists] and I had actually faced off on one of those C-SPAN early morning call-in shows. We were on the opposite side on getting the Iraq war started. We were saying, 'This is a terrible idea,' but we were cordial to one another."

A few months later, says DeMarco, "another great guy," James Standish with the Seventh-day Adventists, told him he should meet a new person with the Southern Baptists, Dr. Barrett Duke. Duke was the chief lobbyist, the director of government relations, for the Ethics and Religious Liberty Commission, the public policy arm of the Southern Baptist Convention, which is the governing body for the sixteen million Southern Baptists. He "understood our issues immediately," DeMarco says. "He understood that smoking kills unborn fetuses when pregnant women smoke. He understood the broader health consequences of smoking, and he says, 'We need to be involved in this.'" Sosa makes a critical point: "Barrett sees the consistency, in that they are pro-life people, and that if you're going to be pro-life, this is a definite pro-life issue." Sosa also credits Duke with understanding that theirs was an issue through which the Southern Baptists could "earn credibility for other issues that they may be more isolated on."

Barrett Duke engaged his boss, Rev. Dr. Richard Land, president and chief spokesman for the Ethics and Religious Liberty Commission, who turned out to be an equally passionate believer in tobacco control. Within a year, the commission had passed policy positions that built on and broadened a number of tobacco-related policies that they had adopted during the 1980s, such as calling upon their members to stop growing tobacco.

Not surprisingly, some public health advocates resisted aligning themselves with religious conservatives. Some feared that they would thereby be giving respectability—innocence by association—to extreme views. Some gay and lesbian members of health advocacy groups felt uncomfortable working closely with fundamentalists who viewed them as bound for hell. Yet most health advocates welcomed the clout of the conservative Christians in an alliance against the power of the tobacco lobby.

Among the resistant was TFK president Matt Myers, who says at first he harbored doubts, not only about the goal—a network of national faith leaders willing to rally their members behind tobacco control—but also about DeMarco's ability to achieve it. The first few times he met DeMarco, Myers was convinced that "there's no way" a man with such strong progressive views on such a broad range of issues "can be in a room with conservatives, let alone conservative religious people, and not get into a war." He also felt that "the rumpled, frenetic, slightly disheveled way he goes about life" wasn't a fit either.

Then "you see Vinny in a room with a group of leaders who run from progressive, more modern religious leaders to the most conservative Bible-reading leaders, and he moves back and forth as seamlessly as it's possible to do—and in genuine friendship. It comes down to people trusting and having faith in him."

What helps build that trust and faith, Myers has decided, is that DeMarco doesn't allow himself to get sidetracked by the issues on which he disagrees with people he is working with. He doesn't let those issues get in the way of his relationship with them or in his organizing and working with them. One of the reasons Myers thinks that people trust DeMarco is because "when Vinny sits down and works with you on an issue, he's working with you on *that* issue. It's genuine. It doesn't matter that he disagrees with you on ninety-nine other issues. And it doesn't *feel* like he disagrees with you on ninety-nine other issues."

For a while, even with the Southern Baptists on board, DeMarco continued to reach out to conservative faith groups without much more success. Finally, he realized: "Southern Baptists, sixteen million. I don't need more than that. The important part of the Southern Baptists is that they are fully engaged; tobacco control advocacy has become one of their top priorities."

11

Faith in Action

Between 2001 and early 2009, DeMarco reached out to his national faith partners, with TFK's Patricia Sosa, to mobilize state faith leaders across the country to join existing state health advocacy efforts:

Whenever I am asked to help out in a particular state or city, I send out an e-mail to all of the national faith leaders and ask them who they have in that jurisdiction that can help us. Then, I do follow-up calls, starting with Rev. Clayton Childers from the United Methodist Church, who almost always provides me with names of local United Methodist clergy or lay leaders who are eager to help and often form the backbone of our local organizing group. For example, Clayton referred me to Revs. Glynden Bode in Texas and Dee Stickley-Miner in Ohio, both of whom played critical roles in faith outreach work in those states. Other national faith groups, including denominations like the Seventh-day Adventists, Jews, Muslims, Southern Baptists, American Baptists, the United Church of Christ, Lutherans, Episcopalians, and Presbyterians, and interdenominational groups like the Health Ministries Association, Church Women United, the Woman's Christian Temperance Union, and the International Parish Nurse Resource Center, have all helped us to find local leaders.

During these years, DeMarco and Sosa helped state and local faith and health alliances through every phase of their development, toward the goals of stronger smoke-free laws, higher tobacco taxes, and, at the least, no drop in funds for state tobacco control programs. The two over time would bring together local faith and health leaders in Virginia, Wisconsin, Minnesota, Oregon, Colorado, New Jersey, Connecticut, Ohio, Montana, Kansas, Oklahoma, Indiana, Kentucky, North Carolina, Pennsylvania, Texas, and the District of Columbia, among others. They organized several regional meetings of faith and public health advocates and national experts as a cost-effective, cross-pollinating organizing strategy. Often, the TFK team itself organized the meeting, led the outreach to make sure of attendance (lots of phone calls and e-mails), developed the agenda, recruited the experts, and took responsibility for the follow-up.

In the process, they would troubleshoot. In 2004, the city of Columbus, Ohio, passed a smoke-free workplace ordinance, and the opposition succeeded in placing on the ballot a referendum to have it repealed. The ordinance was in jeopardy, and local leaders asked DeMarco to help mobilize the Columbus faith community. He put together a press conference with dozens of local faith leaders, who urged voters to support the smoke-free law. They did so, and, in part inspired by Columbus, the entire state of Ohio soon became smoke free.

DeMarco and his TFK colleagues sometimes engaged in direct advocacy to link ideal messengers with receptive decision makers, as when they recruited Seventh-day Adventist national leader Dr. DeWitt Williams to meet with his old friend and fellow Adventist, Mayor John Street of Philadelphia. DeMarco's weekly report included the result: "They are very interested in working with us on a major push for a clean air law in Philadelphia with a strong push from the faith community. We have another call with them scheduled for next week." Philadelphia became smoke free.

As in DeMarco's Maryland campaigns, every event he and his TFK colleagues helped plan had a built-in media component, and each media initiative had multiple objectives—especially toward stimulating outreach, organizing, and delivering an advocacy message to decision makers. For each event, the TFK team—including TFK's communications specialists—would be fully engaged in providing media advocacy tools: media advisories, press releases, and even video news releases. They helped organize press conferences and cultivated and followed up with local TV producers and journalists. They also made sure that occasions planned by others—the many "faith breakfasts" and special events such as a February 14 "Show Your Love" happening in Indianapolis—became media worthy.

Creating Something from Nothing

One lens through which to view the contributions of DeMarco and the TFK team to state tobacco control efforts is the nature of their support for one state over time. A good example is Indiana, for several reasons. To begin with, when the TFK team first offered help in 2003, Indiana had a well-funded and expertly directed state tobacco control program that faced a politically powerful threat to its funding. Yet its voluntary health organizations in the

1990s had failed to create a vibrant tobacco control movement to stand behind the state program or advocate for more. As a result, and to compound this failure, no one—neither government agencies nor private foundations such as The Robert Wood Johnson Foundation—was willing to invest in infrastructure for tobacco control advocacy in Indiana.

Also in 2003, there were exemplary individual tobacco control leaders and strategists in Indiana. Most impressive among them was Karla Sneegas, a public health official with many years' experience and deep commitment to tobacco control advocacy. In that rare convergence of the right person in the right job, Sneegas since 1999 had headed Indiana's statewide tobacco control program, Indiana Tobacco Prevention and Cessation (ITPC), initially funded by the state attorneys general settlement with the tobacco companies. TFK's Peter Fisher; its Midwest regional coordinator, Aaron Doeppers; and its research director, Danny McGoldrick, were frequent visitors to Indiana, Sneegas says, helping set up ITPC and helping advocate for money. Patricia Sosa was particularly successful with ITPC's outreach to the Indiana Latino community.

In addition to building a $33 million program from scratch within the bureaucracy, however, Sneegas had constantly to confront the downsizing political funding habits of the Indiana legislature and successive governors. "We'd had a decent amount of funding," says Sneegas, "and then suddenly the lieutenant governor—running for governor—and powerful legislators eager to divert the funding to their pet projects were just coming in and doing slash and burn." At that point, Sneegas reports that DeMarco showed up and said, "Let's build a faith coalition." Her perception is that "somewhere along the way, filling the void of not having a stand-alone functioning health coalition, it morphed into a faith *and* health coalition."

In Sneegas's view, a key DeMarco resource was his national faith network connections. For instance, when he came to Indiana for a planning meeting of the developing coalition, Sneegas says, he set up "a meeting with the key person from the Episcopal Church here, who had been connected from his Episcopal contact at the national level. There were probably four or five connections like that that were made." Then came DeMarco's follow-up, as Sneegas observed it: "There would be a face-to-face meeting; then there would be very important e-mail that he would do after that, encouraging them to become a part, thanking them for everything they were doing. He would team them up and introduce them, sometimes to me, sometimes to Aaron, sometimes to the Methodists' Dan Gangler, who was the co-convener, and he made that *web* happen. Vinny created that. And then you were—*boom!*—you had them at the table."

DeMarco's weekly updates on TFK's work in Indiana between 2001 and

2007 outline exactly how this happened. The reports yield more than organizing nuggets; they relate sustained organizing and technical support over time that draws upon much of the learning, and many of the innovative techniques, that DeMarco was testing through his serial campaigning in Maryland—adjusted to the Indiana advocacy landscape.

If not the comprehensive plan DeMarco would craft in Maryland when he was leading a campaign, reports reveal a sequence that consistently repeats—from planning to outreach, organizing to mobilizing, action to victory, as well as celebration, thanks, local leadership development, advocacy renewal, and refocusing. Reduced to their essence, the techniques that worked in Indiana were:

> Unrelenting outreach to potential new allies, one-by-one, through incessant networking, including cross-pollination through the national faith, labor, and other networks
>
> Resolution after resolution as a prime organizing tool
>
> E-mails, one on one and through distribution lists; conference calls; meetings—to plan, to teach, to embrace new members, to allocate assignments, to build trust and cohesion, to inspire and energize
>
> Events: faith breakfasts, press conferences, a candidate's forum, a holiday event, celebrations, campaign launches
>
> Media advocacy: no event without a media advocacy plan; cultivation of reporters; media advisories; releases, including video news releases; op-ed pieces; letters to the editor; newsworthy national speakers
>
> Action: dissemination to decision makers and the media they pay attention to of tailored resolutions demanding specific executive or legislative action; lobbying; barrages of letters and postcards; nonpartisan election campaign demands on candidates; candidate letters and postcards
>
> Fund-raising for TFK's state work and for the Indiana activities, both 501(c)(3) and 501(c)(4)

The words and phrases that most often appear in DeMarco's reports are, not surprisingly, "called," "organized," "talked to," "followed up," "got people to come," "conference call," "met with," "attended meeting," "drafted," "prepared." There is also his characteristic embrace of coworkers: "YEAH PARISH NURSES!!!" "WE LOVE THE PARISH NURSES!" "What a pleasure it has been to work with Patricia on this event and on our other faith outreach projects!!! She did a great job of MC'ing the event and making opening remarks on Friday night that really motivated people!" Of his TFK field colleague, Aaron Doeppers, who is *not* a clergyman, DeMarco exults, "The Right Reverend Doeppers spoke eloquently (after doing a great job of helping organize)!"

Indiana Leadership Development

State and local advocates complain that technical support by national groups is invariably evanescent: experts are sent in, add advocacy heft for a while, and then leave. They do nothing to help develop the indigenous leadership needed to sustain progress. On this count, DeMarco's Indiana reports absolve TFK of this gap in their support: one recurring theme is the nurturing of such leadership—out of both need and desire.

In his report for the week of December 8, 2003, for example, DeMarco describes a planning meeting at a conference in Boston that he attended with Karla Sneegas and Aida McCammon of the Indiana Latino Institute. Their intent was to reach out "to United Methodist churches in January and possibly focus on a different denomination every month. We will be having a conference call about this on Wednesday." By the week of January 26, 2004: "Aida McCammon is taking a leading role in coordinating the faith work there. She reported on our call that they already have a couple of dozen faith groups signed on to their resolution." The week of February 9, 2004: "Patricia and I also spent time meeting with Aida McCammon of the Indiana Latino Institute who is playing a leading role in organizing the faith outreach work in Indiana."

In another instance, the leader recruited was a local parish nurse. The week of November 8, 2004, DeMarco reports: "Patricia, Pete, Aaron and I worked on trying to find an organizer to help mobilize the faith community; particularly for the Valentine's Day event we have planned. I spoke with a local parish nurse leader who might be interested and we set up a follow-up call for Monday." Less than a month later, DeMarco reported spending "a substantial amount of time working with Aaron on setting up our new arrangement with Pat Thorlton, a Parish Nurse leader from Clarian Health, who will be coordinating the faith outreach work in the state. Pat has brought other staff at Clarian Health into the project also."

In the same December 6, 2004, report, another local leader makes an appearance: "We had several conference calls with Pat, Aida and Patricia from the Indiana Latino Institute, and Dan Gangler from the United Methodists to continue making plans for the February 14th event. Pat and her staff put together a great invitation letter and Dan has arranged for it to be signed by the United Methodist Bishop and a top UCC [United Church of Christ] leader. The letter will be going out during the first week in January to the about 250 faith groups that have signed the Hoosier Faith and Health Resolution as well as to over 1600 other congregations in the Indianapolis area."

Thereafter, Pat Thorlton's name recurs with "her staff" in event planning and follow-up mobilization in support of funding for ITPC. Dan Gangler's name also appears with greater and greater frequency. Another local leader, Johnny Kincaid, shows up in the January 9, 2006, report: "We have finalized the leadership team of the Coalition: we will have two Co-Conveners, Dan Gangler of the United Methodist Church representing the faith community, and parish nurse Pat Thorlton from Clarian Health representing the health community, and, in addition, Johnny Kincaid from Evansville will be a liaison to local organizations. We think the leadership team will be very effective." Effective it must have been. "Finally, we are going to help our local leader United Methodist Dan Gangler get to the APHA [American Public Health Association] meeting in Boston," DeMarco writes in October 2006, less than a year later, where Gangler was receiving an advocacy award for which Karla Sneegas nominated him. That's leadership development.

DeMarco is diffident about his role in Indiana. Aaron Doeppers, TFK's Midwest coordinator, is diffident about his own role but not about DeMarco's: "We built the Hoosier Faith and Health Coalition [HFHC] to fill advocacy holes in an existing larger advocacy plan—and in that more focused role, HFHC was probably as strategic as anything Vinny ever did as just a role player rather than the center of the movement. There has been great crossover into the wider tobacco advocacy effort resulting from HFHC work—Reverend Gangler and a couple others have become tremendous additions to the wider advocacy efforts and coalitions."

It is true, however, that while DeMarco and Doeppers helped develop indigenous Indiana leadership, such leadership never fully replaced the TFK role. Doeppers says in-state leadership has grown by fits and starts, and he and DeMarco continued to play leadership roles in HFHC. Although they recruited co-chairs from health and faith groups and nurtured local leadership, Doeppers says, "Vinny really was the personality center of the effort from the start, regardless of my involvement or who the co-chairs were." He and Doeppers set the strategy for the group, and DeMarco was the de facto leader in the coalition's incarnation. The two of them worked with key members of the group "on a consensus basis." Still, Doeppers and DeMarco pushed specific strategies, for example, HFHC's first big faith advocacy event, which they suggested that the coalition sponsor and that TFK funded via a grant to one of the HFHC member organizations. The coalition's pledge drive with individual churches, Doeppers says, "came directly from Vinny's experiences elsewhere"; then "the locals embraced the vision we urged, we all shaped it together, and for the most part the locals made it successful." Over time, then, Doeppers and DeMarco gradually yielded leadership to the emerging local leaders.

In early 2008, Karla Sneegas reflected on the technical support (not her term) that Indiana received from DeMarco and his TFK colleagues. "Vinny's a bridge builder. Our health folks don't really understand how to build bridges.

But how much more can you achieve when you bring religion together with health—especially in a state like Indiana, where there's not a lot of diversity to begin with? Could somebody else have organized the way that Vinny organized in Indiana? Maybe. But his ability to mix it all together, connecting and networking, is so rare."

Pressuring Congress

DeMarco's inspiration for organizing national faith leaders in Faith United was their ability to lead TFK to their affiliated state leaders and to encourage their state colleagues to get involved in tobacco control. Partly because this effort originated in DeMarco and Sosa's work with TFK's state support team, it had not at first occurred to TFK's leadership that the support could flow back to D.C.—that once organized, state faith leaders could be of help to TFK's federal lobbying team. By 2005, that oversight was corrected.

A brief historical detour: In 1998, when DeMarco's MCI was building momentum for a one-dollar cigarette tax increase, TFK came close to achieving its highest legislative priority in Congress: comprehensive FDA regulatory authority over every aspect of cigarette manufacturing and marketing. Through a suspect early-twentieth-century legislative sleight of hand, tobacco products had been expressly exempted from FDA regulation, and the tobacco lobby had easily kept it that way ever since. Now the tobacco industry, fearful of lawsuits brought by all the state attorneys general and of bankruptcy from massive punitive damage awards against them, agreed to accept comprehensive FDA regulation of all tobacco manufacturing and marketing in exchange for an annual cap—in the billions of dollars—on any such awards. The companies, the state attorneys general, and national voluntary health organizations led by TFK signed a formal agreement to support the congressional legislation needed to make this happen. In the spring of 1998, in a rare bipartisan effort led by Senator John McCain, then chair of the Senate Commerce Committee, the committee by a nineteen-to-one vote sent a bill to the Senate floor that was measurably stronger even than the agreement. It enjoyed the full support of President Clinton and Vice President Gore.

Two months later it was dead—in no small measure done in by furious tobacco industry lobbying and the industry's $50 million saturation advertising blitz against the McCain bill. (Readers interested in the ins and final outs of this legislative cliff-hanger may want to look at my book on the failure of the settlement, *Smoke in Their Eyes: Lessons in Movement Leadership from the Tobacco Wars* [Vanderbilt University Press, 2001]—a lugubrious counterweight to this book.) DeMarco said to me at the time: "What the tobacco control people don't have with them is the force of the United Methodists fully mobilized!" Much less, the force of the entire faith community.

Renewing this battle was not on the to-do list of the new president, George W. Bush (or of his closest political advisor, Karl Rove, a former tobacco industry lobbyist). Nor was it on the agenda of the aggressively pro-industry Republican congressional leadership, in particular the House majority leader, Tom DeLay—propelled into politics as a regulation-averse pest exterminator. Nevertheless, through the first few years of the Bush presidency, the TFK federal lobbying team kept the candle lit, especially with members of Congress. But DeLay, by far the most powerful force in the House, had been boasting to his tobacco industry friends that he alone had sidetracked the FDA bill in the House in 2004 and would continue to do so until hell froze over. By 2005, TFK's lobbyists had generated a small head of steam in the Senate and were trying to launch a more vigorous campaign.

They had marveled at the power of the state faith and health coalitions to effect policy change at the state level. Their potential for helping the FDA campaign was self-evident. Working closely now with TFK's federal lobbying team, DeMarco and Sosa organized a letter from all the national faith leaders to every member of Congress—including, of course, DeLay—expressing their united support for FDA regulation of tobacco. DeMarco was amazed that when they "asked the Southern Baptist leader Dr. Land to send a personal letter to DeLay, he did."

Why expend all this effort on such an intractable foe? Patricia Sosa and Capitol Hill veteran Anne Ford, the Senate lobbyist for TFK, agree that a politician like DeLay needs, as Sosa says, "to understand that his position is not in keeping with the views of people in his district. And the religious community, which [DeLay] publicly says he's close to—that he's not listening to them either." At the time, she says, after the 2004 elections, their goal with DeLay was "to get him to not be so active—maybe give him a little bit of pause."

The Faith United leaders kept up the pressure, not only with letters, but also with events, including a national press event to celebrate TFK's 2006 annual Kick Butts Day, featuring Faith United's national spokespersons, the Methodists' Winkler and the Southern Baptists' Land. This event marked DeMarco's first meeting with Rev. Land. "The first words he said to me were, 'You know, Vinny, I wanted to put in my speech that the tobacco company executives have cloven hoofs. But my people wouldn't let me, they took it out.'" That event made TFK's staff and leadership even more committed to encouraging the involvement of the faith community, Ford says, because "it was clear that the faith leaders at the event were committed and they were *engaged*. All three of the representatives of the religious groups were fabulous speakers, [using] compelling prophetic language regarding the toll of tobacco and why regulation is so important." As she stood with TFK president Matt Myers and executive vice president Bill Corr, the three agreed, "It just doesn't get any better than that."

2007: A New Congress, a New Opportunity

In January 2007, with the Democrats now in control of Congress, the Faith United leaders sent a new version of their letter to all the members. Tom DeLay was gone in a cloud of corruption. In his place, two former Maryland legislators had ascended to the Democratic leadership of the House of Representatives: Congressmen Steny Hoyer, as majority leader, the second most powerful post in the House, and Chris Van Hollen, the new chair of the highly influential Congressional Campaign Committee.

DeMarco could now open the door to the House leadership for TFK. In early October, he arranged for Patricia Sosa; Grayson Fowler, TFK's House lobbyist; and himself to meet with Hoyer's chief of staff, Terry Lierman. They were joined by the majority leader and "made the pitch directly to cosponsor the legislation." Next, DeMarco met with Van Hollen, who said he would do all he could to get them more cosponsors and to get them a vote as soon as possible on the FDA legislation. Van Hollen was especially interested, DeMarco says, in highlighting the broad faith community support for the legislation among Democratic leaders.

The bill for comprehensive FDA authority over tobacco still faced one steep legislative hurdle: the very real threat of a veto by President Bush. The House Democrats would not be a problem (with a few tobacco-state exceptions). But the FDA bill would need enough votes from Republicans to gain the two-thirds majorities required in both the House and Senate to override a Bush veto, and here the Southern Baptists had their greatest influence.

At first, TFK focused on mobilizing Faith United's state advocates. For example, TFK's lobbyists identified virtually the whole congressional delegation from Tennessee, a tobacco state, as likely nay votes. But Tennessee produces not only tobacco but also strong faith communities, and the delegation needed a loud wake-up call from their most congenial—and powerful—constituents. As in other states, this effort would involve exhaustive outreach and organizing, tasks that fell largely to DeMarco and Sosa. In early 2007, they drafted and arranged for a letter on the FDA legislation to go out from Tennessee faith leaders to the Tennessee congressional delegation. The letter's signers were a diverse group of twenty-six, including three prominent Southern Baptists (among them, Dr. Land himself, who was based in Nashville), several prominent leaders in United Methodist Men and other Christian denominations, Jewish leaders, and the Parish Nurses. American Cancer Society leaders in Tennessee delivered the letter directly to Republican senator Lamar Alexander.

In the late summer of 2007 in Nashville, the Reverend Land opened a press conference in support of the FDA bill. "When you have a figure like Dr. Land, the media will come," says Sosa. "ABC, CBS, NBC, Fox. We had the *Tennessean*, an AP reporter, NPR. I think we got all the major broadcast outlets. Dr. Land not only spoke, but stayed and answered questions." Dr. Land was there again and again when DeMarco and Sosa needed him to join in an action to support the FDA bill: taking part in a planning conference call, headlining a media event, challenging recalcitrant members of Congress, praising Republican members who cosponsored the FDA bill, testifying before Congress, cosigning a letter to the Democrat and Republican leaders or to all members of Congress, putting his name to an op-ed piece in a wavering legislator's hometown newspaper, and visiting—lobbying—key members. Similar coalitions of faith leaders sent letters to key senators and House members across the country.

When Grayson Fowler, the TFK lobbyist charged with building support for the FDA bill, made the rounds of congressional offices, he told the legislative assistants, "We've got everybody from the Sikhs to the Southern Baptists," as he handed them an information packet that included a letter signed by all the faith groups and, at Senate offices, a copy of Dr. Land's testimony. "That just so registers with members of Congress," Fowler says, "you don't really have to say any more. Half the time, they don't even look at the letter. They get the point that there's a broad spectrum of faith support for this legislation. And that takes us to a different place—particularly in conservative Republican offices, which have a tendency to view the public health community as radical." Liberal members, says Fowler, "could think, 'Dr. Land doesn't support us on virtually anything. Why should we listen to him?' But most liberal politicians feel this is an *opportunity*, not an impediment—an opportunity to build a relationship. Supporting what Dr. Land calls for on tobacco makes it more difficult for liberals to be characterized as being anti-faith or anti-religious. It's a great opportunity for Republicans, too, because voting with the Southern Baptists gives them cover with their anti-regulatory business allies."

How Odd Fellows Work Together

For DeMarco, Sosa, and their TFK colleagues, did the deep divide on social and political issues between them and political and religious conservatives create a barrier to their close collaboration on tobacco? DeMarco feels they all "understand each other a little bit better. For me, personally, prior to working with them, if you had mentioned to me evangelicals or Southern Baptists, all I could think of was that these were the same people who elected George Bush, the people who have done all this horrible stuff. Now, I think of Barrett Duke—a wonderful guy! That's been very important to me." Sosa says they found common ground in humor. "We laughed every time we got together." When the conservatives got a judicial appointment through, she and DeMarco "were very polite every time. We said, 'Oh, Barrett, I'm sure you're happy.' And he looks at us and says, 'Well, I'm sure you're not happy!' It's understood: we work on tobacco exclusively. They know where we are; we know where they are."

The working relationship that has evolved between the TFK team and the Southern Baptists, especially Barrett Duke and Dr. Land, illuminates our understanding of a sensitive advocacy alliance and accompanying technical support. As we have seen, the foundation laid for this collaboration is deep commitment to clearly demarcated common objectives, within which mutual respect and genuine affection can take root despite great philosophical and political differences.

A Rare Bipartisan Achievement

As the 2007–2008 FDA campaign heated up, the teams shared their political intelligence—and lobbying assignments. For instance, TFK's Senate lobbyist, Anne Ford, said the Southern Baptists told the TFK team who they thought Senator Edward Kennedy should approach regarding cosponsorship of the FDA bill on the Republican side. It was their help, Ford said, that made the *very* conservative Texas Republican senator John Cornyn feel more comfortable about taking a role as a leading cosponsor. DeMarco finds himself marveling at a later strategy session in Senator Cornyn's office, in which he was surrounded by Dr. Land and Cornyn's conservative staff: "We had a great conversation about the Southern Baptists' and Senator Cornyn's support for the FDA regulation of tobacco legislation. But, when they talked about other issues on which I certainly did not agree with them, I was thinking, 'What am *I* doing here?!'"

The help was not all one way. DeMarco played the principal liaison role, going back and forth between, for instance, the Southern Baptists' Duke and the TFK team with questions and tasks. Then, among themselves, the TFK team would parcel out the time-consuming but critical backup tasks for the faith leaders—drafting and editing of letters, testimony, press releases, and press advisories of upcoming events. TFK's communications specialist, Nicole Dueffert, says she went to the early events at which Duke or Land spoke, then would "take his testimony and turn that into kind of a speech for our press conference." She and DeMarco provided background and other advocacy materials on the bill but recognized and respected the fact that the religious groups would do their own evaluation of the bill and make their own arguments for supporting it. Ford makes clear that it was best for the Southern Baptist lobbyists to go alone, without the TFK lobbyists, because they had their own relationships with legislators: "That was better because they bring a different perspective to the table and it also demonstrates to the members of Congress and their staff just how much *they* care about the issue."

Of particular importance, DeMarco believes, is knowing where to draw the line between "what you can ask *them* to do and what *you* have to do." Specifically, "Barrett Duke, Jim Winkler, Dr. Williams from the Seventh-day Adventists, Barbara Baylor from the United Church of Christ—they all feel very strongly committed, but *they* don't want to organize an anti-tobacco campaign. They all have other priorities, but they love to be part of the tobacco control campaigns. But we do the work."

The breadth of the effect of Faith United Against Tobacco was manifest July 30, 2008, when the FDA bill gained a veto-proof 326-to-102 majority in the U.S. House of Representatives, a majority that included half the House Republicans. But President George Bush threatened a veto, and the bill never came to a vote in the Senate in 2008. In 2009, however, with a supportive Barack Obama as president, both the House and Senate passed the legislation by large bipartisan majorities. On June 22, 2009, in a celebratory Rose Garden ceremony, President Obama signed into law the FDA omnibus regulation of tobacco. Faith United Against Tobacco leadership was represented in the front row by its chair, Jim Winkler. Also there were Baptist Bishop Doug Miles, United Methodist leader Rev. Cynthia Abrams, Muslim leader Dr. Sayyid Syeed, Seventh-day Adventist leader Dr. DeWitt Williams, and Southern Baptist leader Dr. Barrett Duke.

"To Vinny's credit, he created a national coalition to support the FDA bill that is real," says TFK's Patricia Sosa. "There are a lot of people that are able to put coalitions on paper that are very impressive. This was a coalition with a backbone."

Faith Happens

The success of Faith United Against Tobacco destroyed a myth invented by the tobacco industry but fearfully embraced by tobacco control advocates at the dawn of the tobacco control movement in the 1960s that labeled church groups as "neo-prohibitionists," motivated by faith, not science. To avoid being discredited by the same label, scientists and health professionals, along with the voluntary cancer, heart, and lung health associations, largely shunned close collaboration with faith groups. With the shibboleth shattered, the tobacco control movement had tapped into a new source, not only of political power, but also of internal spirit.

No one had anticipated the effect that embracing the faith community—and the DeMarco factor—would have on health advocates. The veteran health lobbyists, at first not at all convinced that DeMarco's wooing of the faith leaders was a productive strategy, have become true believers. TFK lobbyist Grayson Fowler tells of a time when the TFK team couldn't get access to several congressional offices, including those of some Democrats, "because they're so used to hearing from the public health community year in and year out on this issue. But Lerone Allen goes into their office and she's a Seventh-day Adventist, a religious representative, she's African American. It's a totally different look for them. She gets appointments. She gets them on as cosponsors. She's done a fabulous job. And she does it with—excuse the expression—religious persistence."

TFK staff attitudes have changed in parallel ways. Victoria Almquist, who has been with TFK almost since its creation in the late 1990s, commented that during the early years, staff members simply assumed that all their colleagues were political liberals and secular—and they would often make comments based on this assumption, to the discomfort of the one or two staff members who, indeed, were neither. DeMarco and Sosa's faith outreach, Almquist observed, has changed that. Several new valued people with conservative religious and political orientations now work on the TFK staff.

Karla Sneegas, the veteran health advocate in Indiana, reflects on the effect that DeMarco's efforts to bring the faith and health communities together in her state has had on her health colleagues and herself: "Faith leaders, whatever their religious philosophy, seek a greater good for the world. And that sense of a greater good was felt by everyone drawn into our Faith and Health Coalition. And it is exhibited in every aspect of Vinny's work. In every way that he goes about mobilizing and organizing, the greater good is honored. We've always said, 'Tobacco is a bipartisan issue,' but we didn't act as if it were a bipartisan issue. This is actually *living* that it is a bipartisan issue. Because when you bring different religious factions within, it really is."

Part IV

Lessons in Strategies and Leadership

Vincent DeMarco is no revolutionary; he's not even a radical. He does not pretend to have the key to long-term fundamental systemic change, such as a Canadian-style single-payer health-care system that every disinterested, sober expert agrees would be vastly superior to what we have now; or the nationalization of the tobacco industry, which David Kessler as FDA commissioner argued is the only way to tame the tobacco demon. Nor can DeMarco help much in confronting those issues that deeply and evenly divide us: immigration, gay marriage, abortion, or the redistribution of wealth through more progressive taxation.

DeMarco's skills and strategies come into play where there exists broad, generalized popular voter support for policy change that the power of threatened interests has thwarted. Under such conditions, DeMarco goes about mobilizing and focusing that public sentiment into a political force capable of counteracting the power of the lobbies. While DeMarco may not be a political radical, he undertakes these campaigns in ways *radically different* from those that most progressive issue advocates have grown accustomed to, whether or not they have proved effective.

The DeMarco Way

DeMarco has done most of his work in Maryland, a comparatively wealthy state, predominantly Democratic in its politics. The state has a relatively strong labor movement. It has a large urban culture. It has diverse communities of faith, some of which have been historically active in policy advocacy, individually and collaboratively. It has had progressive newspapers both covering and weighing in editorially on the campaigns DeMarco has waged.

Thus, it's fair to ask whether the strategies DeMarco developed in Maryland have much to teach advocates in other states, or in countries with greatly differing social and political structures and traditions. We have only part of the answer to this question when we looked at the success of his strategies in other states and in Congress through his work with TFK. After all, it would be harder (though DeMarco thinks not at all impossible) to get the Southern Baptists who were indispensable in much of the tobacco control wars to join the ranks of other progressive social justice campaigns such as health-care reform. Yet the short answer to how much these strategies have to teach advocates in other places is: *a lot*. Especially useful are the comprehensive advocacy campaign planning, the boundary-stretching organizing, the integrated and relentless media advocacy, and the focus of campaign energies on elections before lobbying.

The Nine Questions

As I suggested in the introduction, one way to gauge the general applicability of the DeMarco techniques is to compare them to a proven method of strategic planning for policy advocacy campaigns, the Nine Questions developed by Jim Shultz of the Democracy Center. The questions continue to evolve, with variations, over time. With Shultz's permission, I describe the Nine Questions here, taking some liberties but essentially naming them as he conceived them. Questions 1 through 5 look outward at the political and media environment within which the policy campaign must be waged. Questions 6 through 9 look inward at the development of a political force strong enough to overcome the external barriers it is likely to encounter.

Looking Outward

Question 1. Objectives: What do we want now? If an advocacy campaign is to achieve anything significant, the question "what do we want now?" often turns out to be the single most important, time-consuming—and difficult to answer—of the Nine Questions. This is not a question about what we want ultimately—however important a grand, long-term vision is—but what we want *right now* (although still bearing in mind what we want next, and what we want ultimately). Is this near-term objective significant enough, yet realistically achievable in the short term, to fully engage the energies of supporters?

Question 2. The target audience: Who has the power to give us what we want? Who has the power to make what we want happen, and who has the power to stop it from happening? This means those who have constitutional power (for example, governors, legislators, and, at election time, voters). It also includes those who have real power—formal, if not constitutional—such as the elected majority leadership of each legislative body, committee chairs, and indeed, all legislators.

Question 3. The messages: What do they—the holders of power—need to hear? Moving these different audiences to act requires crafting and framing a set of messages that will persuade each of them to do what we want each to do. Although we must always root these messages in the same basic campaign themes, we need to tailor them differently to different power holders, depending on what each will respond to. In most cases, advocacy messages have two basic components: an appeal to what is right, and an appeal to the power holders' self-interest.

Question 4. The messengers: From whom do the power holders need to hear the messages? To know each of the power holders well is also to know who has particular influence with them. To whom are they politically indebted and responsive? Whom are they most eager to please? Who intimidates them? (To whom are they financially indebted?) Whom do they trust? respect? honor? fear? like? perhaps even love? Who are the staff members who have their ear and trust? Who are the lobbyists they have grown comfortable with? The same message has an entirely different effect depending on who communicates it. Who are the most credible messengers for each audience? In some cases, these messengers are experts whose credibility is largely technical. In other cases, we need to engage the authentic voices who can speak movingly from personal experience.

Question 5. Delivering the messages: How can we get the power holders to hear the messages? There is a continuum of channels through which to deliver advocacy messages to the power holders. These range from the personal (for example, lobbying) to the confrontational (for example, protest action). The most effective means available to citizen advocates without either special access to the power holders or vast financial resources is often media advocacy, that is, approaching the mass media strategically as indirect channels to the power holders.

Looking Inward

Question 6. Taking stock: What have we got? Campaigns generally don't start from scratch but build on existing strengths, so an effective advocacy effort begins with taking careful stock of the advocacy resources already there to build on. This includes inside and outside leaders, past advocacy experience, networks and alliances already in place, and staff and other organizational or allied capacity, information, and political intelligence.

Question 7. Filling gaps: What do we need to develop? Identifying the advocacy resources we need that we don't have means looking at alliances that we need to build or strengthen, networks we need to expand, and capacities such as outreach, media, and research, which are crucial to any effort. What kind of technical support do we need and where can we get it? And, inevitably, money.

Question 8. First steps: How do we begin? What are our most effective first steps? How do we begin to build now toward ultimate legislative action?

Question 9. Strategic flexibility: What do we do when the plan isn't working, runs into unforeseen roadblocks, or confronts unanticipated opportunities? As do any travelers on a long journey, campaign organizers need to check their course at every stage. They need to reevaluate strategy, revisiting each of these questions (Are we aiming at the right audiences? Are we reaching them? Are we building the support we hoped to build?). They remain open to the need to adapt their plan and their campaign to new events, shifts in inside and outside personnel, and change in general.

About Part IV

DeMarco does not consciously ask these Nine Questions in the form that Shultz asks them. Yet, in the next three chapters, we will see that his strategies and tactics answer each question as each campaign begins and unfolds—so clearly that an advocate who has read the case studies in Parts I, II, and III of this book could design and implement an issue campaign, readily putting DeMarco's strategic innovations in place by following the Nine Questions planning method.

In Chapter 12, we examine how DeMarco goes about providing answers to the first four "looking outward" questions. Chapter 13 examines how DeMarco's strategies respond to the fifth question, focusing on lobbying and media advocacy. Chapter 14 assesses DeMarco's strategic response to the four "looking inward" questions.

Chapter 15 turns toward campaign leadership. DeMarco is unique in many ways, yet there are replicable campaign leadership lessons to be drawn for aspiring campaign leaders, especially in recognizing their own leadership strengths and acknowledging what missing leadership roles they need to reach out to others to fill.

12

Before We Do Anything Else

Some forty years of involvement in issue campaigns—mostly consumer protection or public health—have taught me that one of the most common strategic errors passionate advocates fall into is leaping before they are ready. "There oughta be a law!" "Let's run a public education campaign!" "Let's attack the special interest lobbies!" "Let's go lobby!" "Let's create a coalition!" I understand these impulses, but they may prove useless sound and fury unless the activity they generate grows from a coherent plan that answers first questions first.

Question 1. Objectives: What Do We Want Now?

Most advocacy groups know generally what they want, that is, they know their ultimate goal: preventing tobacco use, reducing gun violence, providing universal health care. They also usually have a keen sense of the specific policies that will help them get there: spiking cigarette taxes—and hence prices—high enough to discourage teenagers from buying cigarettes, limiting handgun sales, transforming a notoriously defective health-care delivery system into a workable universal health-care system. But too often they turn at once to "campaign mode" without first taking the time to test and refine long-term and short-term objectives. A quick bill drafting and they're off to lobby.

How long might it take to find out what we want now? Some members of DeMarco's coalition did not want to wait two years to answer this first question. They were restless; a few were mutinous. All had signed a resolution calling upon the state to provide exactly what their campaign slogan implied: Health Care for All Marylanders. Many who had been fighting for universal health care for years thought they knew the best way to get there, in theory, including Peter Beilenson, who had recruited DeMarco, and many of the health-care experts at Johns Hopkins. Early on, DeMarco himself tended to agree with them. What would work best was a single-payer system combining the best elements of the prevailing systems in every industrialized country but ours. Yet it was three years into the campaign before the coalition released its proposed health-care plan, and then it wasn't a single-payer plan.

Even abandoning the single-payer plan for a less radical prescription for universal health care did not assure the continuance of a powerful coalition. The nonspecific framing of DeMarco's original Health Care for All! resolution was enough to gain more than twenty-one hundred signatories. The specific plan the coalition finally adopted drew eleven hundred signatory groups, more than enough to constitute a viable political force.

If an advocacy campaign is to achieve anything significant, answering the question "What do we want *now*?" is at least as critical as answering the question "What do we want eventually?" because it is pragmatic. It must offer realistic hope for legislative success in the short term. As DeMarco has demonstrated, in the process, we can apply several developmental tests to such short-term objectives.

1. What we want next must have the potential to serve as an effective election campaign issue. The very first—the threshold—question DeMarco asks before he embarks on any full-scale legislative campaign is, Does what we want next have the potential to serve as an effective election campaign issue? His threshold act is funding a well-designed poll that answers this question. He needs the poll to show not only whether a substantial majority of voters supports the objective, but also whether a significant number care enough to change their vote based on the stands of competing candidates for state elective office, regardless of party. In 1997, DeMarco's poll showed such public support for a cigarette tax increase, even one as high as $1.50. In 1999, the poll demonstrated strong voter support for health-care expansion—though not if it meant giving up current health insurance. This was enough to determine DeMarco's willingness to proceed with a health care for all campaign, and to make him wary of a single-payer solution.

2. Our proposed legislation must reflect what we want, appeal to the allies we will need, and retain those already with us. In the early 1990s, the tobacco control coalition in Maryland consisted almost entirely of public health advocacy organizations. They sought a one-dollar cigarette tax increase, a goal they lacked the breadth of support to achieve. By contrast, in forging his 1997–1999 $1.50 cigarette tax increase campaign, DeMarco painstakingly constructed a new alliance of forces with the political clout to overcome Bruce Bereano's tobacco lobby, tax-averse broader business lobbies, tax-phobic Republicans, and conservative Democrats. He engaged faith leaders on the basis of the dreadful health effects of tobacco use on their congregants, and he secured the allegiance of other core partners by drafting, with their participation, an organizing resolution promising to allocate funds to their priority programs.

The Fair Share bill gained traction because it split the business community. It enjoyed the passionate support of Wal-Mart's competitors, beggared by having to pay into the state fund that provided health care for Wal-Mart's workers. Although the Chamber of Commerce and other business groups opposed the bill, many in the business community remained neutral: Wal-Mart's fight was not *their* fight. Had the coalition stuck with the part of the Health Care for All! bill that mandated *all* businesses, small as well as grand, to provide worker health-care coverage, the business lobbies would have successfully united in opposition behind the leadership of their ally, the Republican governor.

3. The current political structure and environment must offer realistic hope of success. Choosing the next legislative objective requires deep analysis of the current political environment. The worthiest policy goal backed by the strongest grassroots coalition cannot make headway without potent inside leadership, and without at least neutralizing enough potential inside opposition.

The starkest illustration of this imperative in DeMarco's campaigns was the drastic change in short-term objectives required by the upset election of anti-health-care expansion Republican Robert Ehrlich as Maryland governor in 2002. Instead of the second-stage campaign for the Health Care for All! plan spearheaded by the supportive Kathleen Kennedy Townsend, DeMarco faced a determined foe of any such plan. The question could no longer be, "What do we want, given Governor Townsend's leadership and advocacy?" Revised, it became, "What can we get that can be a step toward health care for all, keep our coalition engaged, and override the opposition of Governor Ehrlich?"

The answer came in two packages. First, the coalition continued to pursue its Health Care for All! bill, especially in the Maryland House, where support for health-care expansion was strong. Even though "no health care went anywhere," coalition members could see some fight and enough progress to keep them engaged. Even better, the coalition devised interim policy objectives it hoped to achieve, not by confronting the new governor but by circumventing him.

Sometimes, the calculus of what to propose comes down to intimate knowledge of the political and *personal* predilections of only a few key legislative power wielders. Intelligence provided by DeMarco outposts at the state capitol in Annapolis, such as lobbyist Len Lucchi, as well as DeMarco's own days and hours walking the capitol halls, led to a crucial decision in 2007 to abandon a core objective of the cigarette tax/Medicaid expansion campaign that year: that the legislature dedicate the tax increase to funding Medicaid expansion.

The shaping of an advocacy group's legislative objective also can be influenced by the principled, unprincipled, or merely stubborn resistance of a *single* power holder capable of blocking the path to enactment. This was the case during the 1998 trial run for the MCI cigarette tax increase, when the chair of the Senate Budget and Taxation Committee, Barbara Hoffman, wanted her committee, not a rigid legislative formula, to allocate any tax proceeds. As a result of her opposition, in 1999, DeMarco convinced almost all his partners that there was no politically viable alternative to stripping the allocations for spending from the coalition's bill.

Sometimes the political calculus requires not a change in the desired legislation, but nonaction on the part of a campaign. Unless Senate President Mike Miller got enabling legislation for slot machines, he would—and could—block *any* new health-care initiative, including health-care expansion. So DeMarco made sure that the Health Care for All! Coalition stayed, as he put it, "aggressively neutral" on the slots issue, despite his own and most coalition members' distaste for slots. He feared that any action at all could derail the delicate balance of the governor/House/Senate leadership compromise that traded cigarette tax/Medicaid expansion for a statewide referendum on slots.

4. *The objective must be large and appealing enough to mobilize the energies of the engaged, but not so radical as to drive away the moderates.* Utopian grandiosity is a nonstarter, and so is thinking too small. In planning his next incremental health-care campaign in 2006, DeMarco, still facing a hostile Republican governor, seized upon the element of the Health Care for All! bill that would increase the cigarette tax to help fund Medicaid expansion. He recognized that although the proposed increase of thirty-six cents was attractive as part of the grand Health Care for All! scheme, standing alone it was too small to energize the coalition. He determined to pursue a one-dollar increase—enough to expand Medicaid to fund every uninsured parent in Maryland up to a level above the poverty line, but not too grandiose to drive away the moderates.

Like the painful decision to abandon the reach for single-payer health care, this choice was another application of what DeMarco and Schneider call the Rule of the Thirds—keeping the Rabid Third engaged, without driving the moderate Middle Third away.

5. *If achieved, the short-term objective must be a step toward the ultimate goal, not a detour or roadblock.* When the election of Ehrlich in 2002 thwarted DeMarco's grand plan to achieve health care for all Marylanders, he mostly did not look for compromise with the conservative governor (except for one prescription drug discount bill that Ehrlich signed and Governor O'Malley sought to implement). Instead, as just noted, he chose to pursue collateral objectives that circumvented the governor's power. Yet by focusing on these objectives

to answer the coalition's question for 2003, What do we want *now*? DeMarco was able to redeem his vow "to go forward, not backward." Only an informed and shrewd reading of the state's political environment and decision-making structure made that possible. Throughout the ten years of short-term health-care campaigns that DeMarco organized, he never undermined the ultimate objectives embodied in the original Health Care for All! plan.

Another instance: Gaining in 1999 only a thirty-cent cigarette tax increase instead of the one dollar targeted, DeMarco bided his time. In 2007, he achieved a one-dollar cigarette tax increase in the Health Care for All! campaign. When the issue is dollars, not the structure of a government program or regulation, one significant gain does not preclude another later.

Finally, Medicaid expansion in 2007 did not radically change the existing health-care system, but it did expand government-financed health-care coverage to tens of thousands of uninsured Marylanders and was a major step toward the goal of quality affordable health care for all Marylanders. The single-payer advocates did not see it this way. One told DeMarco that he would oppose Medicaid expansion because its passage, by filling a dramatic hole in the health-care safety net, would weaken support for a single-payer system. In their fervor, the single-payer advocates would have missed what could yet turn out to be a step toward the goal of universal health care, whether or not actually run by the government.

Question 2. The Target Audience: Who Has the Power to Give Us What We Want?

With a concrete campaign objective set, DeMarco addresses questions of power. He maps not just who has the power to make the campaign's objective happen, but who has the power to stop it from happening. This informs not only the shaping of the legislative objective, but also the scenario of the entire campaign.

There is a civics-class answer to the question of who has the power. Although the governor has the authority to propose and to veto legislation, only majorities of the House and Senate have the power to enact legislation. Voters, as DeMarco never forgets, have the constitutional power to elect and not elect governors and legislators—but only on Election Day.

Constitutionally, some governors are stronger than others. Maryland has a strong governor with ample power over budgets—meaning the funding or starving of legislators' cherished projects. That power enabled a determined Governor Glendening, in 1999, to force the Maryland Senate finally to swallow a cigarette tax increase that it didn't like. Great power is formally, if not constitutionally, also vested in the elected majority leadership of each house—in Maryland, the speaker of the House and the Senate president. Senate President Mike Miller haunted DeMarco's dreams through several campaigns and then led the fight for DeMarco's Fair Share bill that made the difference in getting the bill passed. House Speaker Mike Busch made Medicaid expansion happen.

Citizen campaigns, especially where passions run high, have a tendency to go public with a brassy launch without checking to see who's got the big guns. Sometimes there is a supportive inside leader in the legislature with the power and the commitment to achieve a campaign's objective quietly. At that moment, a media attack or a well-publicized action alert might arouse opposition. It might annoy that leader. It might be a waste of always scarce human and financial resources.

This was the case in March 2008, as the Maryland legislature wrestled with a vast and growing budget deficit and Senate budget cutters proposed to delay the funding of the Medicaid expansion plan just enacted in the Special Session at the close of 2007. Ready to launch a media blitz in protest, DeMarco checked with Kristin Jones, chief of staff to House Speaker Busch, an unwavering supporter of the Medicaid expansion. The delay "will not happen," she told DeMarco, "and media uproar will not help." A politician's "trust me" is almost never a pledge to lean on. Its worth depends on which politician with what power to keep what promise, as well as that politician's past commitment to the issue and track record in fulfilling pledges. In this case, Busch, as the strong House speaker, met all the tests. He had the power, and DeMarco had reason to trust both Busch and his chief of staff. He held back on going to the media. By contrast, as the budget shortfall cost-cutting pressure built, Jones blessed DeMarco's release of a poll that showed that Marylanders did not want to have health-care reform cut back, backup that strengthened the hand of supportive leaders in the House and Senate. While dozens of cherished state programs were slashed, and despite the wishes of some in the state Senate, the landmark Medicaid expansion proceeded on schedule.

Finally, with regard to legislative and executive power, in 2008 two-thirds of the U.S. House of Representatives voted for the bill to grant the FDA authority over tobacco marketing, and three-fifths of the senators *cosponsored* the bill, in no small measure the direct result of pressure from Faith United Against Tobacco. When President Bush threatened a veto, however, the bill died. But on June 22, 2009, an enthusiastic President Obama signed the bill into law.

Next on the power continuum—and on certain issues sometimes even more powerful than the top three positions, especially in blocking the paths of bills to the chamber floor—are the committee chairs and the ranking minority committee members. Sniffing out where true power resides requires a far more artful political analysis than simply looking at who holds what office. Some nonranking members of the legislature are powerful because they do their homework, can be relied on, and are therefore respected—and followed. Others may do the same but are arrogant, or showoffs, or personally disliked. Paragons of virtue with sweet dispositions may have crossed the House speaker or Senate president; choose one of these as your leader, and your bill could perish out of mere spite.

Every legislative campaign must have inside leaders in each house: bill sponsors whose sponsorship carries weight with many, and ideally with both liberals and conservatives; respected cosponsors whose names signal to different constituencies that the bill is worthwhile—and politically safe; openly or quietly supportive committee chairs who enjoy the trust of the House leadership, like the Maryland House Health and Government Operations Committee chair Peter Hammen and Speaker Busch. It's also important to avoid recruiting legislative pariahs as cosponsors (though the primary sponsor can't deny them), whose names as cosponsors could only be exploited by opponents. Knowing who holds the formal and informal leadership roles—and the pariahs to avoid—tells DeMarco much he needs to take into account in shaping his legislative strategy. He took great care in recruiting the House and Senate sponsors of the Health Care for All! bill. Note, too, the tireless cultivation of legislators whom he knew to have influence with the House speaker or Senate president. And note how his final campaign objective to secure the 2007 one-dollar cigarette tax increase and Medicaid expansion was tailored to the needs, both political and personal, of the two powers he needed to placate most, Governor O'Malley and Senate President Miller—having secured the firm support of the third great pillar of power, House Speaker Busch.

Is there a difference between power and influence? Look at legislative staff members, who have no formal power. They are often young and easily underestimated. If they are not close to the committee chair or member they work for, they may have neither influence nor delegated power. If they are close, knowledgeable, and trusted, they can wield great influence.

Do lobbyists have power? Influence leaches into power when a lobbyist's close friendship with a legislator is larded with campaign contributions and a list of favors done. Tobacco lobbyist Bereano held such power, sufficient for him to claim truthfully that, in 1997, "we had that thing dead in the water." The campaigner needs to know how well-connected lobbyists will affect a member's actions. Those actions may be as subtle as a bill's nominal sponsor displaying less than maximum effort to recruit more sponsors or to press hard for a timely vote. DeMarco, the lobbyists who work closely with him (Len Lucchi and Eric Gally), and his inside allies (legislative veterans like Chris Van Hollen) understand these sensitive power vectors, since they live them.

Civic groups have influence that can ripen into power. Compare the Smoke Free Maryland Coalition, which in 1997 had not much power and little influence, with the greatly expanded and powerful MCI in 1999, with politically weighty new partners such as the teachers' union. The SEIU that waged a fierce campaign for the Fair Share bill also exercised its fearsome political power. The use of its monetary resources to develop and publish ads decrying the failures of named legislators was surely a forceful incentive to others not to cross the union.

DeMarco's drive to enlist the clergy in campaign advocacy speaks to their special power—call it moral power or the more mundane power of a politically responsive flock. Bishop Miles once erupted in frustration at the Baltimore City Council's reluctance to enact a cigar tax, vowing that ten thousand parishioners would vote their outrage in the next elections—that's a threat backed by power. DeMarco puts it more delicately: "The moral authority of faith leaders—just because they are who they are, policymakers have to listen to them. They can't ignore them. They don't have to do as the faith leaders ask all the time, but they have to at least be listened to." The cigar tax passed.

Question 3. The Messages: What Do They— the Holders of Power—Need to Hear?

Some advocacy groups have a spontaneous sense of what they want to say to power holders, and they sometimes give in to a compulsion to scold, shake, lecture, plead with, and whine at the power holders who are not doing what they should be doing. This does not often persuade the objects of the advocates' indignation or open a constructive dialogue. Other advocacy groups, such as medical societies or unions, need the power holders, especially governors and legislative leaders, over time for favorable action and even leadership on a wide range of issues that are a priority for them. They feel that they need to ingratiate themselves with the power holders, avoiding confrontation, demands, and unpleasantness. They speak softly and do not carry a big stick.

DeMarco, however, asks not what he or his allies feel compelled to say, but what the power holders need to hear to persuade them to do what he wants them to do. He speaks softly for a while, but he does not hesitate to unveil a club to gain the attention of those to whom civil messages never penetrate. To divine what messages will move what power holders, and when, requires political, personal, and even psychological understanding of *each* key power holder. This means drawing upon the best intelligence obtainable on what motivates each power holder, and only then determining what buttons to push, and what line of argument, what evidence, or what potential threat or reward is most likely to move that person to right action.

Before undue cynicism engulfs this discussion, I hasten to point out that there are many legislators who share the worldview of the advocates, and who awake each morning *not* asking themselves, "What can I do to advance or defend my career or my power today?" Instead, as longtime Maryland committee chair Maggie McIntosh observed of House Speaker Mike Busch, every day he asks himself, "What can I do today to help the people of Maryland?"

A Mike Busch or a Maggie McIntosh needs to hear a message that begins, simply: "Here's a problem you care about. Here's a solution that will help. Here's solid evidence that it can work. Here's what you can do to make it happen." But even a saintly legislator, of which there is not likely to be a majority, needs to hear other, more politically relevant messages, including ones like these:

> Taking on this issue, leading the fight, or even just voting for it, will not be a suicide mission. Large majorities of voters (especially in your district) support this solution. In fact, they support it so strongly that they will be even more inclined to vote for your reelection—and against any election challenger who fails to support it. Here's the evidence.
>
> You will not be alone. Other leaders you respect, who share your values, are with us in this battle.
>
> There is a broad, deep, strong, *bipartisan* coalition to support you in this effort, with resources to carry the fight to the media to generate popular support.

Even these reassuring messages are not quite enough. Politicians generally want to be appreciated. At a workshop on social justice advocacy in Maine several years ago in which a number of veteran advocates participated, the question came up, "Should we thank politicians who do the right thing?" Ralph Nader's sisters, Claire and Laura Nader, said: "No. They are merely doing the job they were elected to do. That should be reward enough." At that point, another participant, the attorney general of Maine, Jim Tierney, a courageous trustbuster and consumer protector, stood up and said: "Look, I'm a politician, and I'm like other politicians. We want to be loved, not just by our family and close friends, but by strangers, hundreds, even thousands of strangers. We need to hear that we are loved, over and over again." So power holders need to hear a contrapuntal chorus of messages: science, reason, argument, appeals to *their* core values, hymns of praise, or, at a dead end, threats of retribution. DeMarco would shamelessly seize any opportunity publicly to hail governors and legislators who turned his policy goals into enacted laws, no matter how hard it had been to get them there.

So much for the elected officials. What of the voters, who also hold power—the power to initiate, continue, or end the term of elected officeholders? What messages do voters need to hear? In DeMarco's plans, voters are the very first power holders to address. His premise is that the power holders who control the state agenda in the legislature will rarely budge unless the power holders who hold the keys to *their* power are prepared to use them.

Voters need to hear the following one or two years before the next state elections:

> The initiative is important to *you* and to people you care about.
> The solution offered makes good sense and will help solve problems you are concerned about.
> A serious citizen coalition of organizations you belong to or admire is forming to fight against special interests opposed to this solution.
> Community groups are flocking to the initiative—don't let your group be left behind.

Next, the summer before the election, they need to hear:

> A campaign now under way to get legislators to pledge their support to this initiative serves your interests and concerns.
> *Then*: These candidates have signed the pledge, and these others won't sign it.
> *Then*: Here's why you need to vote for those who signed the pledge and not for the others.

The focus then shifts to legislative power holders. The governor needs to hear:

> The voters who voted for and support you want this objective. They want it strongly, now, and undiluted. This is why you got elected. Even many voters who never supported you want it.

The legislators need to hear:

> Those who opposed this initiative lost their seats; pay attention, so you don't lose yours.
> Anyone who sides with the special interest lobbyists (for example, Big Tobacco) is voting against the will of the voters.

To those legislators who signed the pledge: Keep your word. The voters are watching.

Finally, the postfilibuster message should be:

There are painful political consequences for those who would thwart the will of the people.

Question 4. The Messengers: From Whom Do the Power Holders Need to Hear the Messages?

As the *Baltimore Sun*'s Fraser Smith noted in contrasting the influence of the tobacco lobbyists with that of the Smoke Free Maryland messengers: "The smoking foes have few personal relationships with committee members. Personal relationships are the coin of the realm in Annapolis. Veteran lobbyists have been full-service friends to senators or delegates they sometimes refer to as 'votes,' vacationing with them, handling a divorce, playing golf and advising on legislation."

To know the power holders well is also to know who turns them off: officious, condescending, grating public scolds; political enemies or rivals; their supporters, whom they don't want to be seen taking orders from or even being responsive to (this applied to DeMarco himself as his public profile grew); anyone too predictable; anyone too humorless. For example, in cataloguing the missteps of the Smoke Free Maryland Coalition in the 1997 legislative session, Smith also noted that although the coalition "packed the House and Senate committee hearings with celebrity witnesses, . . . the anti-smoking team was almost too democratic, including witnesses and gimmicks that annoyed committee members. [Among them were] two young men who have been proving for years that youths can buy cigarettes in vending machines."

DeMarco, by contrast, learned through each successive campaign more and more about those whom key lawmakers listen to in the privacy of their offices, and made sure he developed relationships with them. One striking illustration he recounts is the tug-of-war between two crucial messengers to former governor William Donald Schaefer, who was serving as state financial comptroller during DeMarco's 1997–1999 cigarette tax campaign. The campaign needed Schaefer's endorsement to offset the argument of the tobacco lobby that raising the tax would send hordes of smokers across the border to buy cigarettes in low-tax Virginia, cutting into Maryland tax revenues.

Tobacco lobbyist Bruce Bereano was close to Schaefer. DeMarco was not, but he was a friend of Lainy Lebow-Sachs, whom he saw as the voice of

Schaefer's good angel. "While Bruce tugged Schaefer in the pro-tobacco and pro-business direction, Lainy always pushed him to do things like fight for gun control and other social justice causes," DeMarco says. "I spent months meeting with Lainy to convince her of the importance of the tobacco tax effort to reduce teen smoking, and when she was convinced, she helped me reach out to Schaefer." In the end, Schaefer listened to Lebow-Sachs on the tobacco tax, not to Bereano.

By contrast, during the run-up to the 1999 legislative session, DeMarco went aggressively public with the messages of the tax increase campaign. He organized town press conferences around the state, with a roster of speakers chosen to resonate with both the political culture and the power structure of each town and its legislators.

The Clergy, God's Messengers

The clergy are DeMarco's favorite messengers, we now know, but he calls upon them selectively, depending on the audience. Among the most ubiquitous are the United Methodists, of whom Bernie Horn observes: "They will send a message from their bishop down. They are a very large denomination. They have very strong social beliefs. They have committees that do public policy. So they are actually set up to be a powerful political force."

In Philadelphia, working to persuade the mayor to lead a forceful push for a clean indoor-air law, DeMarco and his TFK colleague Michael Berman learned that both the mayor and one of his top advisors were active Seventh-day Adventists; they made certain that both heard from their Seventh-day Adventist constituents. In Indiana, as DeMarco and his TFK colleagues were organizing pressure on key state legislators not to cut the state's successful tobacco prevention and cessation program, they helped mobilize the Southern Baptists in the northern part of the state, where they had a strong presence, and the Methodists in other districts. As DeMarco and Patricia Sosa sought conservative Republican support—or only nominal resistance to FDA regulation—they turned again and again to Dr. Richard Land, the political spokesman for and temporal embodiment of the conservative Southern Baptists.

When the mostly Episcopal and Presbyterian clergy in Maryland, representing mostly middle- and upper-class congregations, held back from endorsing a steep cigarette tax increase out of sensitivity to the regressive effect of the cigarette tax on low-income smokers, it was the eloquent Bishop Douglas Miles to whom they listened. Of the many in his congregation who were indeed smokers and poor, he spoke of the disproportionate health devastation of smoking to them and his hope to spare future generations from smoking through the cost barriers created by higher taxes.

Sometimes the very breadth of faith community support served as the message. In the fall of 1998, at the height of the Maryland primary campaigns, almost all the members of the Central Maryland Ecumenical Council appeared at a press conference for the $1.50 cigarette tax increase and the election pledge campaign. Later, during the general election season, DeMarco unloaded the most politically pointed attack of the entire campaign: the paid ad calling dramatic attention to the Republican candidates' indenture to the gun, tobacco, and gambling lobbies ("Bang! Cough! Ka-ching!"). The ad was introduced as "a message from the Interdenominational Ministerial Alliance." Not only was the ministerial alliance the right messenger on the health and moral issues raised by smoking, but also it was the most credible nonpartisan messenger in a cacophony of politically partisan voices. Similarly, when lobbying the U.S. Congress in support of FDA regulation of the tobacco companies, TFK's lobbyists were delighted to open their conversation with: "This bill is supported by faith groups from the Sikhs to the Southern Baptists."

The Business Community

DeMarco learned during the campaign for the Fair Share bill that business owners could be among the most effective spokespeople for the need to make quality health care affordable for all. They were especially effective as credible messengers for the message that it was unfair to make businesses that responsibly provided health care pay for those that didn't. Taking this lesson further, DeMarco announced in the spring of 2009 that two Maryland local chambers of commerce—the Greater Baltimore Black Chamber of Commerce and the Black Chamber of Commerce of Anne Arundel County—had both endorsed his health care for all plan. And several of the Maryland business owners he recruited to work on his statewide campaign became national spokespeople for federal health-care reform, taking their case directly to President Obama himself and to his director of the White House Office of Health Care Reform.

Authentic Voices and Stories

Among the most newsworthy and persuasive messengers throughout DeMarco's campaigns were people who could highlight the personal effect of the public health problems he was trying to solve, for example, widower Joel Lapin and his public testimony about how tobacco addiction—and tobacco industry lies—killed his wife, Marsha. And in his Health Care for All! campaign, DeMarco distributed widely a compelling booklet put together by Sarah Penna, social worker and Open Society Institute–Baltimore Community Fellow, called "Faces of the Uninsured," which compiled the stories—broken down by county—of more than 140 Marylanders from across the state who suffered from lack of health insurance. No American's story and voice could be more authentic than that of Sarah Brady, wife of President Reagan's press secretary Jim Brady, who was permanently crippled by bullets meant for the president. Sarah Brady not only brought both media attention and authenticity to DeMarco's gun control campaigns, but she extended the reach of her effect to DeMarco's 2007 tobacco tax campaign with her testimony as a smoker and survivor of lung cancer.

Children's Advocates—and Children

As DeMarco shifted the identity of the cigarette tax campaign in 1997 from Smoke Free Maryland to MCI, he recruited five core partners in addition to the faith community whose very names communicated that this campaign was about children, especially the teachers' union. The public trusts teachers when they speak of the needs of children. Teachers have firsthand knowledge of the factors, such as seductive tobacco advertising, that sap their students' independence. Furthermore, teachers' unions are politically potent when speaking to legislators.

Children themselves are authentic voices; their youth dispels the reflexive distrust many members of the public feel toward adult advocates. In a town meeting and press conference in Howard County leading up to the 1999 legislative session, DeMarco deployed a cross-section of legislators, cosponsors of the bill, and role models for their fellows in the legislature, but not as the lead spokespeople. These were teenagers, whose credibility framed the story in the October 3, 1998, Howard County edition of the *Baltimore Sun*: "Kicking off a grass-roots campaign for a $1-a-pack increase in the state cigarette tax, Howard County activists employed a new weapon yesterday in their battle against the tobacco industry: children."

Health-Care Professionals

Throughout his campaigns, DeMarco relied on doctors, nurses, hospitals, and other health-care professionals to make key points about public health and health-care expansion. Within Smoke Free Maryland, DeMarco drew heavily upon MedChi, the state Medical Society, on issues of tobacco and health, because when it comes to questions of health science, doctors are among the most credible messengers. They are not always the most *effective* messengers, however, for many physicians are more used to dictating than to persuading. An arrogant doctor testifying on the health effects of smoking and the merits of a policy proposal may have scientific credibility but can still turn off legislators.

One on one, however, the right doctor can be a most effective messenger to a legislator. American Medical Association lobbyists cherish their most valued weapons, which they call their "golden bullets"—the doctors close to each member of Congress in every congressional district: the family pediatrician for younger members; the geriatrician for older members, along with their cancer, heart, or lung specialist. Pediatricians generally are more effective with liberals; male surgeons tend to appeal to social conservatives. The dual credibility of a doctor who is also a public health official, such as Peter Beilenson when he was health commissioner of Baltimore, influences legislators.

Policy Experts

Sometimes an outside expert can be effective as the voice of authority. Having produced a richly ecumenical gathering of local clergy for the faith leaders' press conference just described, DeMarco was delighted when the July 14, 1998, *Baltimore Sun* added weight to the occasion by calling upon a veteran tobacco control advocate, Boston law professor Richard Daynard: "[Daynard] said that as far as he is aware, the involvement of the religious groups in the anti-tobacco movement has been limited to resolutions passed in annual conventions and the divestment of tobacco stock by many denominations."

Outside experts can often do the best job of laying to rest specific concerns on legislators' minds. TFK research director Danny McGoldrick and his deputy, Eric Lindblom, both knowledgeable on every scientific question related to tobacco health effects and policy, proved effective witnesses in Maryland and other states—especially as they were experienced and sensitive enough never to talk down to legislators. In these circumstances, local experts, however qualified and diplomatic, might be scorned as the proverbial prophets in their own country. There are exceptions: in his health-care campaigns, DeMarco has been blessed by the special standing in Maryland of Johns Hopkins University health policy experts—viewed by many Maryland legislators as both awesomely expert and locally attuned. Dr. Alfred Sommer, then dean of the Johns Hopkins Bloomberg School of Public Health—a highly regarded physician, a policy research expert, a warm and engaging speaker, *and* local— proved an invaluable spokesman. National expertise came into play to establish the soundness of economic projections that predicted the fiscal responsibility of the Health Care for All! plan, when DeMarco chose the expensive, Washington-based, scrupulously neutral Lewin Group to stamp the data as unimpeachable.

Where experts are coming from philosophically or politically can greatly enhance their credibility. DeMarco goes to great lengths—and expense—to engage Republican pollsters and conservative economists when he is seeking to persuade conservative legislators. When, in 1998, he commissioned a poll that demonstrated that even Republican voters supported the cigarette tax increase bill by 58 percent in favor to 30 percent opposed, he enlisted a blue-ribbon Republican pollster to coauthor the study. It was this pollster whom the *Sun* identified and quoted.

The Medical Society, itself a credible messenger, hosted the August 12, 1999, event announcing the first Health Care for All! campaign poll, a gathering that included a mix of outside experts. The society's president was conspicuously present and spoke to the press, a breakthrough that reflects, as DeMarco notes, the shift in the medical community: "Years ago, doctors were against this, but they don't like the HMO system." But it was Hopkins's Dean Sommer who earned the prize quotation in the next morning's *Baltimore Sun* story by M. William Salganik and Diana K. Sugg: "'Our present health care system is an embarrassment,' declared Dr. Alfred Sommer, dean of the Johns Hopkins School of Public Health. Of 27 developed countries, he said, only three don't guarantee every person health insurance—Mexico, Turkey and the United States."

13

Delivering the Messages

The work of the campaign begins in earnest with the answer to Jim Shultz's fifth question—How can we get the power holders to hear the messages? The effort to answer this question strategically is the essence of the campaign. This is the most challenging arena, and this is where DeMarco invests his greatest effort, once his organizing is well under way.

Lobbying—Direct and Indirect

In-person communication from the right messenger is often the most effective way to deliver a message. This is especially so when the content of the message is political. Thus, a whispered word from a trusted pollster that polls show that the candidate's stance on a bill entails grave political risk can change that stance more effectively than can a front-page story on the same poll; no candidate wants to be *seen* as blowing in the wind of the opinion polls rather than relying on his or her conscience.

DeMarco is a lobbyist, and among his closest colleagues in many of his campaigns has been lobbyist Len Lucchi. Eric Gally, chief lobbyist for the American Cancer Society in Maryland, has also long been a key player in DeMarco campaigns. Though DeMarco devotes much effort to direct lobbying himself, he is at least equally likely to tap his network of allies to find exactly the right person to sway a wavering or unhappy power holder. When he was pressuring Governor Parris Glendening to sign the campaign pledge to support the cigarette tax increase as he had promised, for example, DeMarco reached out to the governor's communications director, "our biggest advocate" inside the governor's staff. Glendening finally announced that he would sign the pledge but kept DeMarco waiting for weeks to get the signed document to him, so DeMarco called upon another ally, the head of the teachers' association, who was close to the governor and could say bluntly to him, "Would you *give* Vinny the paper!" DeMarco got the signed pledge.

To persuade all the gubernatorial and legislative candidates to sign that pledge, DeMarco earlier had relied not on private lobbying but on the very public strategy styled on the Boston Tea Party and waged through the mass media; the candidates saw that their alternative was to get tossed metaphorically into Baltimore's inner harbor. The pressure would come from the broad media coverage of the rally, and the personal and political embarrassment to those who had not signed. The governor got the message, promised to sign the pledge at the last minute, and was hailed as a hero at the rally.

Media Advocacy

A strategic approach to the mass media as a potent weapon in advancing an advocacy agenda is an essential element of every DeMarco campaign. He spends a lot of time thinking about how to most effectively use what he calls this "telephone" to the public. Citizen advocates, who seldom have the same access to lawmakers as have moneyed interests with influential lobbyists, see media advocacy as indirect lobbying, a necessary if imperfect surrogate for *real* lobbying.

Media advocacy, however, has its own strengths. The media have influence. "Media effects" researchers, most prominently political scientists Shanto Iyengar and Frank Gilliam, make a strong case that extensive media coverage signals to people what is important and greatly affects legislative agenda setting, the priority an issue receives from both voters and policymakers. When Marylanders express the feeling that health care is a top priority issue, their opinion doubtless reflects the drumbeat of media coverage on the plight of the uninsured and underinsured, which heightens people's sense of health insecurity. DeMarco's campaigns demonstrate how media coverage can also prime and reinforce citizen mobilization, so that the constitutional power of citizens to elect or un-elect governors and legislators can become a focused political force. The mass media deliver a message that everyone hears, and part of the message to legislators is that *everyone* is listening to and watching you.

DeMarco's campaigns typically proceed in planned stages, beginning with a year or two of public education, broadly defined. When the campaign moves into the primary and general election stage, the media advocacy is focused on voter and candidate education; next, in the legislative phase, on pressuring the legislative leaders and members; and in the post-legislative session phase, on thanks or condemnation. Characteristically, DeMarco's 1997–1999 cigarette tax campaign strategy unfolded in six stages, with media advocacy efforts tailored to each.

Framing Stories to Hook Media Attention

Media advocacy practitioner and scholar Lori Dorfman divides media advocacy into framing for access to the media and framing for content that speaks to your intended audience. By *framing for access*, she refers to shaping a story to gain the interest of reporters and editors, muscling out all the other stories competing for their attention and space. By *framing for content*, or framing the messages, she refers to the need for a story in the newspaper or an online blog, on the radio or TV news, to communicate to the intended audience the message that the campaign needs to deliver.

How does DeMarco go about achieving his media advocacy objectives? Here, I focus on what goes into framing stories that attract reporters and editors, that is, framing for access. In DeMarco's step-by-step process for each event, the first step is to frame the event in a way that attracts media attention. For the release of a poll, he says, his frame might be "Marylanders support tobacco taxes." Second, he uses as messengers people in whom the media will be interested, such as nationally renowned pollster Celinda Lake. Third, his team puts together a short media advisory that highlights their message and attractive messengers. Fourth, they spend a lot of time on the phone pitching the story to key reporters, such as the *Baltimore Sun*'s Scott Shane, with whom DeMarco had built a good relationship. Fifth, they find a good location for staging the event; in the case of the cigarette tax increase, "the state Medical Society office worked well," DeMarco says.

These categories—framing for access and framing the message—like so much else in the art of advocacy, often blur. An access strategy like DeMarco's prized political polls may gain media attention as good stories for political reporters, and also contain within them the message that cigarette tax increases are politically popular. Other media access tactics, such as the rally styled on the Boston Tea Party, may create interest, but the intended message has to be coaxed out of the event, in that case requiring a skillful stretch. Let's take a look at some of DeMarco's successful tactics in creating newsworthy stories.

Polls

Time and again, DeMarco's polls demonstrate that voters do not just support his campaign goals, but do so with such intensity that significant numbers say they would change their votes depending on a candidate's position on the campaign's proposal. Political reporters never seem to get enough of such polls. This is especially true when a newsworthy pollster shows up at the press conference releasing the results, such as a prominent Republican pollster who is able to report to Republican politicians (and nervous Democrats) that there is such a thing as a popular tax increase.

Launches

DeMarco launches campaigns with great drama, not just once but many times, under story lines that vary only slightly. A launch occurs with the release of the first poll, anticipating that a campaign will follow; with the recruitment of the first partners; when the campaign takes on a name; when it opens a resolution drive; when it gains sufficient support in a local jurisdiction; when a new or noteworthy partner comes on board; when it adopts a specific plan, such as the health care for all plan; and when it kicks off a primary pledge campaign, then a general election campaign, and then the push before the legislative session opens. Next, a launch accompanies the bill's passage in the house, and then the opening of the campaign for senate passage. DeMarco has more launches than a navy in wartime—and every one merits a story.

Social Math or Creative Epidemiology: Emphasizing the Local

DeMarco extends the newsworthiness of his polls by calculating the poll results by local jurisdiction to tease out the local implications, thereby creating a fresh story for local reporters. This kind of localizing is only one form of what Australian tobacco control wizard Mike Daube labels "creative epidemiology"—working with the bare numbers revealed by research in a way that dramatizes their significance. More mundane advocates call this "social math." Perhaps the most famous example—and for the media ever fresh— is Ken Warner's reworking of solid data on the death toll from smoking. A scrupulous public health economist and a canny tobacco control advocate, Warner, with solid data to prove it, wrote in the October 16, 1987, issue of the *Journal of the American Medical Association* that "smoking kills more people than heroin, cocaine, alcohol, AIDS, fires, homicide, suicide, and automobile accidents combined."

The MCI print ad, "Today, 60 Maryland children will become cigarette addicts," illustrates this social math, reinforced by evocative visuals—the photographs of sixty Maryland children, twenty of whom would "die before their time" from smoking unless prevalence rates declined. From state studies that have worn out their media welcome, campaigns can localize health data for cities and counties to create new stories.

Progress/Momentum

Another favorite DeMarco media access tactic is a variant of social math: progress reports on the growth of a campaign, each proving newsworthy—150 groups sign on, then 367, then 1,000, and then the incredible 2,100 groups that signed on to the broad Health Care for All! resolution. The momentum builds with the news that gubernatorial candidates have signed on; that majorities of primary candidates have signed the pledge; later, that elected state legislators are signers; that county officials have signed on. The headline-worthy numbers keep going: after taking office, eleven newly elected senators wrote to senate president Miller calling for action on the cigarette tax/Medicaid expansion bill.

Events

"Events," says DeMarco, "are very important because they give people a goal. They give people something to strive for, something to build around—and that's where the media coverage comes from, these events." Reporters seem never to get their fill of DeMarco-generated happenings. Among his favorite and most reliable are prayer breakfasts, which combine the general newsworthiness of clergy with the appeal of a singular event. A DeMarco certainty is that media events featuring clergy make sure-fire stories.

The media love youth events, too, which ranged in DeMarco's campaigns from the Boston Tea Party–style rally to youth-led marches on the legislature to the photo of Talbot County students holding the MCI banner, accompanied by a quotation from an eighth grader suggesting that legislators opposed to the cigarette tax increase deserve a grade of F. "Students can make a big difference in the media," Bernie Horn observes, "which is your real lobbying, not walking door to door. The students may not be able to persuade legislators directly, but the media coverage of the students will get their attention."

Holidays and Other Anniversaries

The well-reported rally in Indiana on Valentine's Day—"Show Your Love" (by supporting a cigarette tax increase to save children)—suggests the potential in tying campaign events to an annual holiday or anniversary. In the health-care campaign, DeMarco and Glenn Schneider imagined announcing a thousand resolution signers by July 4, staging the event as a "declaration of health-care independence." (They missed that target but still were able to generate news at the thousand-group landmark.) The Boston Tea Party rally on May 31, 1998, was scheduled to coincide with the World Health Organization's World No Tobacco Day.

Investigative Reports

To throw light, and well-deserved mud, on foes like the tobacco companies, nothing beats the appeal of once-secret industry documents that reveal company executives' perfidy in their own words. When the National Smokers Alliance, billing itself as a "grassroots organization," tried its hand at media advocacy by announcing that its claimed 180,000 Maryland members were outraged at the proposed cigarette tax hike, Glenn Schneider turned the story on its head by instigating an exposé of the alliance as a phony tobacco industry front. He did this without publicly saying a word, simply providing a *Sun* reporter with internal documents unearthed by the state attorneys general in their lawsuits against the tobacco companies. Instead of the story about smokers revolting that the Smokers Alliance had promoted, the *Sun* reported the treachery of the movers and money behind the alliance, "Philip Morris, the largest U.S. tobacco company, and the public relations firm Burson-Marsteller."

Shameless Opportunism

DeMarco knows that if you are opportunistic, with a sharp eye for breaking stories, you can often find a news peg on which to hang a story frame. Most dramatic in the Health Care for All! campaign was the unexpected and unscripted comment to a reporter by Republican governor Ehrlich's interim health secretary, Nelson J. Sabatini, that health care was a basic human right and should be universal. With a governor hostile to health-care expansion newly elected, no one in the legislature was paying any attention to Health Care for All! until Sabatini's remark, when it "leaped back onto the state legislature's agenda," DeMarco says.

To liven up interest in another story with the desired frame, "Coalition Urges Tobacco Tax Hike," DeMarco used as the hook the news that the son of a smoking-addicted World War II veteran had joined the MCI coalition. In yet another story, felicitously headlined "Smoker Owens Backs $1 Cigarette Boost," the spokesperson (and supplemental media hook) was an addicted tobacco farmer who was also a county executive, giving reporters a "man bites dog" news twist.

DeMarco even managed to piggyback on an obituary, though this was not as tasteless as it might sound. On the eve of the primary election in 1998, an emotionally powerful and pointed obituary reported the death of Marsha Lapin, a longtime activist who had contracted lung cancer the past summer and had testified in support of the $1.50 tax. Her September 11 obituary in the *Baltimore Sun* quoted DeMarco, "the executive director of a coalition of 300 organizations working for a tax increase on cigarettes and to reduce smoking among youths," who said that Lapin's "illness affected her body, but not her spirit," and added: "The tobacco industry really has caused a lot of misery; her legacy was that we in Maryland are going to do something about it."

Later, DeMarco relied on Lapin's widower to boost press interest at a rally of students as the 1999 legislative session opened. The *Sun* quoted "Joel Lapin, whose wife had died the previous September of lung cancer at the age of forty-nine. 'Please, for those that love you and for those you love, do two things,' Lapin said. 'Continue your pledge not to smoke and do the right thing: Keep up the good work.'" Lapin also agreed to send a letter to both gubernatorial candidates asking them to sign the pledge, and all major TV stations ran a feature on Lapin and his family's commitment to the tax campaign.

Relentless Repetition

DeMarco is never content with just one or two news stories from a good news peg. Not only does he craft variations on one basic piece of news to achieve multiple stories, but he also tries the same news peg again and again if it fails to generate attention the first time. He released the results of the first poll on a cigarette tax increase no fewer than three times in the fall and winter of 1997. Each time, the media treated the release as fresh news.

When DeMarco and his TFK colleagues helped state advocates organize a press event, they did everything conceivable to get the local press to attend—sent advance press advisories, distributed press releases, made reminder phone calls. In the process they provided all a journalist might need to write the story: fact sheets, talking points, choice quotations, and even, for the broadcast producers, video press releases.

So ubiquitous is DeMarco's presence in the capitol pressroom in Annapolis, Schneider says, the new reporters who have not yet learned what DeMarco can provide them "roll their eyes when they see him coming." Nor is his work done when the legislative vote is over. Schneider recalls that after the last vote late at night in the state Senate in 1999, as the advocates and their legislative allies were breathing a sigh of relief and celebrating, he found that DeMarco had disappeared. He had gone back to the pressroom to make sure the reporters got "the story I want."

One form of preparation for press conferences that DeMarco does *not* do is to coach the speakers: "Unlike others in this field, I never spend a lot of time scripting what everyone is going to say. I rely on having good people speak who know the issue and who are good speakers." This uncommon restraint serves a tactical objective: to enhance the spontaneity, authenticity, and interest of the speakers' words.

Framing the Messages That Work

As DeMarco shaped his 1997–1999 tobacco tax campaign, his "public education" forays carried many embedded messages, not least the connection between high taxes and low teenage use of tobacco—as in the message headline produced by the local press conference in Cumberland, Maryland: "Group Believes Higher Taxes Way to Curb Smoking." But before the organizing of the coalition had even begun, the first press conference of the campaign yielded headlines that embodied DeMarco's message not to the general public, but to legislators: "Poll Shows Support of Cigarette Tax Is Healthy for State's Politicians"; "Poll Shows Cigarette Tax May Help Legislative Candidates." One article began: "Anti-smoking activists will push for a whopping $1.50-a-pack cigarette tax next year, and they warn that lawmakers who oppose them will be displeasing voters." The message frame DeMarco and MCI hammered home was not about the *science* of cigarette tax increases but about their *politics*. The targets of those messages were the legislators who had felt no need to pay attention in 1997, but who would pay very close attention in 1999.

Media advocacy is not an add-on to DeMarco's campaign but an integral part of every strategy. From the first stage of public education to the last post-vote hurrah (or brickbat), earned media coverage, with a tactical sprinkling of timely paid advertising, is DeMarco's cure for legislative lassitude and a countervailing force to the invisible lobbying influence of economic interests.

DeMarco does not have a communications specialist on his campaign staff, though his colleagues, Glenn Schneider and Matt Celentano, became highly skillful at DeMarco's brand of media advocacy. DeMarco himself identifies the messages he needs to strengthen voter volition and legislator support, beginning with the analysis of his polls to identify gaps in public and legislator awareness. He turns to communications experts such as his kitchen-cabinet friends Bernie Horn and Len Lucchi for creative techniques to deliver the messages (including the MCI name itself) and for help in crafting campaign ads. He leans on the communications skills of the TFK team to support media advocacy in the states they work with. He selects resources because they fit into his overall strategic message plan, not because they are available.

The framing of progressive messages has become, in recent years, a topic of research-based counsel to advocates. Bernie Horn has written a sound and highly useful book drawing together some of the most valuable insights from the most prominent of these framing theories (*Framing the Future: How Progressive Values Can Win Elections and Influence People*). Yet DeMarco has paid little attention to communications researchers, other than the practical counsel and creative insights Horn offers. His framing strategies flow from his campaign experience, trial, error, learning, and instinct. In practice, DeMarco's message framing in many ways measures up to the basic teachings of some of the soundest work in the field.

Winning Hearts as Well as Minds

Among the most respected framing gurus is Ethel Klein, a leading scholar and practitioner of political communications. Issue advocates who offer only reasoned arguments on behalf of their policy objectives are doing only half their communications job, Klein says. An effective advocacy message must be "at the same time logically persuasive, morally authoritative, and capable of evoking passion. A campaign message must speak at one and the same time to the brain and to the heart." DeMarco understands and practices this. The print and radio ads that Lucchi and Horn developed during the 1997–1999 MCI campaign meet this multilayered standard well. So do such media advocacy stories as those featuring the pleas of teenagers and even a victim of tobacco-caused lung cancer and her widower.

The campaign spoke to the brain when the poll by Celinda Lake revealed that only a bare majority of voters understood that high taxes actually reduce teen smoking. The radio ad script countered this misperception with facts. The print ad that ran simultaneously spoke to the brain with a data-based statistic, a variant of creative epidemiology, by graphically conveying that sixty Maryland children become "cigarette addicts" every day. The radio ad identified its source as the Maryland State Medical Society, an authoritative voice.

Both ads also spoke to the heart. The voice on the radio ad was that of Kathleen Kennedy Townsend, accompanied by what the script baldly calls "sappy music," speaking not just in her authoritative role as lieutenant governor of Maryland but as "the mother of four school-aged daughters." The print ad addressed the heart with its choice of the emotionally loaded, but scientifically sound, term "addict" and with its depiction of the eventual deaths of children. Both the Medical Society and Townsend, who ends by saying, "The big tobacco companies don't like it, but it's the right thing to do for all of our children," meet Klein's prescription for "morally authoritative voices"—as, of course, do the clergy at so many of DeMarco's media advocacy events.

Appealing to Shared Social Values
Susan Nall Bales, founder and president of the Frameworks Institute, which skillfully integrates academic media effects research into practical counsel, cautions progressive advocates to contextualize specific policy proposals by

first showing the larger goals that connect them to values the public readily recognizes and embraces—such as fairness, opportunity, health, and security. DeMarco does this. For example, with Bernie Horn's guidance, he named his 1997–1999 tobacco tax campaign not the obvious Maryland Tobacco Tax Initiative, but the Maryland Children's Initiative. Wordsmith Horn explains that this choice was "about message framing. When you select a name for a group like that, that's the name that's going to be in the paper every time you're quoted. You get to choose how you're framed, how people see you over and over and over again. You wouldn't want to have a name having to do with tobacco tax, or anything with the word 'tax' in it." For the most part, voters supported the tax increase either because they believed that it would cut down on teen smoking or that its proceeds could help fund children's urgent needs—hence, the Maryland Children's Initiative.

More subtly, in the health-care campaign, DeMarco avoided the term "universal health care," which many polled voters felt threatened their present coverage. He evoked instead the broader value imbedded in the phrase "health care for all." Similarly, when the press began to call the Fair Share bill the Wal-Mart bill, DeMarco was alarmed. They had not developed the bill only with Wal-Mart in mind but with a genuine focus on the fairness of *all* large companies to pay their fair share. So the campaign continued to insist on Fair Share to affirm the basic value of fairness, as distinct from a current and specific state of unfairness.

The names Health Care for All!, Fair Share, and Faith United Against Tobacco also met another framing test posed by Susan Bales: the need to find a "simplified concept" that encapsulates what you want.

But Not Getting Framed

Bales observes that advocates too often focus their media efforts on *responding* to their opponents' arguments rather than setting their own frame; thus, they risk becoming trapped within the opponents' frame. For example, when lobbyist Bereano taunted Smoke Free Maryland advocates for failing to make the connection between "their conceptual case against smoking evils" and the tax increase, he was framing the issue as a debate over the scientific evidence that tax increases reduce smoking—right where he wanted the campaign to stall. Even though the advocates had science on their side, Bereano was canny enough to know that a scientific debate alone could never mobilize a citizen movement. DeMarco knows that, too, which is why his primary message frame for the media in the next tobacco tax campaign was not only the proven health benefits of the tobacco tax, but the political will of the people.

The Rot at the Top

Another useful approach to framing relies on the historic insight of Robert Reich, first illuminated in his 1987 book *Tales of a New America*. There, Reich makes a convincing case that much political change in the United States has taken place because it was framed in one of four compelling myths, or narratives, which he encapsulates as "the rot at the top," "the mob at the gates," "the benevolent community," and "the triumphant individual."

While DeMarco's cigarette tax campaigns supply allies and reporters with fact sheets to answer the tobacco industry's arguments, their main thrust in response to the industry's lobbying and propaganda is to hammer away at "the rot at the top." The targets of the attack are Big Corporate lobbying and its corrupt alliances with governors and legislators who would do Big Tobacco's bidding. We saw this focus in the "Bang! Cough! Ka-ching!" ad and the Glenn Schneider–orchestrated exposure of the National Smokers Alliance as a secretly funded industry front group. Other examples are the ad by Bernie Horn and Len Lucchi, "The Tobacco Industry Is Not Your Friend," and Bishop Miles's repeated excoriation, in his speeches and press events, of tobacco company executives' private scorn for consumers, encapsulated in the documented quotation of one who said, "We reserve that right [to smoke] for the poor, the young, the black, and the stupid."

What about Our Disappearing Newspapers?

How would DeMarco's media advocacy have fared were it not for the *Baltimore Sun* and the *Washington Post*? These great newspapers employed uncommonly attentive journalists, and their editors encouraged broad coverage of DeMarco's campaigns and paid attention to them in their editorials. Yet most advocates in most states do not have newspapers with such commitment and resources to turn to. (And with the downsizing of the pressrooms of even these newspapers, DeMarco and his Maryland allies cannot necessarily rely on them any longer.)

Given the changing media environment, how relevant to most citizen policy advocacy campaigns are these Maryland case studies? This is a good question and one that began to trouble me midway through writing this book. I also became increasingly aware that although DeMarco was at least as active with local broadcast TV and radio station advocacy, which *could* readily be emulated in most cities and states, no written account of his campaigns' successes in these media could begin to convey their essence. So I began to develop, with the skilled production and editing of Jessica Fusillo, the companion DVD to this book, *The DeMarco Factor: Lessons in Media Advocacy*.

Nevertheless, not all the news about newspapers is bad. Among strong papers especially, as print readership erodes, online readership explodes through websites and the vast network of online blogs. One analyst calculates that the online readership of stories and columns from papers such as the *Sun* and *Post* is ten times their print readership. Moreover, although specialty beats, such as education and health, may be curtailed, local political reporting survives, and DeMarco's media advocacy has primarily activated political reporters, though he has also successfully cultivated religion- and business-page reporters for critical stories.

Though technologically challenged, DeMarco has bear-hugged the Internet as an organizing tool. He now has access to an electronic megaphone that instantly disseminates to his large e-mail lists every print or electronic story that trumpets the campaign's progress. Because his organizing principle has been to recruit allied organizations more than individuals, every such e-mail will be resent to each organization's network, posted, and linked on hundreds of blogs. Furthermore, direct online reporting has taken up some of the slack in print news reporting. President Obama directs his messages to YouTube for a sound tactical media advocacy reason. You can bet that other political officeholders, the prime target of any policy campaign, pay attention to the new media because they know or believe that their most actively engaged constituents are assuredly paying attention to them.

The basic tactical media advocacy questions remain what they have always been: What medium does our target audience read, view, or listen to? What medium does our target audience believe its constituency reads, views, or listens to? How do we get our message into that medium? The crucial techniques of media advocacy—getting attention and framing the messages—will need to evolve, but they are no less applicable to the new media.

14

Organizing Plus

At the same time as the campaign strategist looks outward to answer the first five of Jim Shultz's Nine Questions, an unsentimental look *inside* the campaign organization is essential to gauge its strengths and address its weaknesses. Equally unsentimental must be a readiness for midcourse corrections, even radical circumnavigation, if the facts on the ground so dictate. Shultz's last four questions are designed to force such analyses.

Question 6. Taking Stock: What Have We Got?

An effective advocacy effort begins with taking careful stock of the advocacy resources we already have. This includes leadership, past advocacy work that is related, networks and alliances already in place, staff and other people's capacity, information, and political intelligence. We don't start from scratch; we build on what we've got. Let's look at the Smoke Free Maryland Coalition, *before* it reached out to DeMarco. Though bloodied by its defeat on the tax increase in the Maryland legislature, it still could count on significant resources, beginning with the skills and commitment of its staff and including the following:

Its coalition of more than sixty organizations, many with active
constituencies; recognized community health leaders; and most
important, the Medical Society and the well-established and trusted
cancer, lung, and heart associations—a coalition that had already won
significant local tobacco control laws

Seasoned member organization lobbyists, especially the Cancer Society's Eric
Gally

Financial support not only from its members, but also from The Robert

Wood Johnson Foundation, which created and generously funded the
staff infrastructure of the coalition

Substantial technical support from The Robert Wood Johnson Foundation,
directly and indirectly, through the national TFK campaign

"Science, truth, and moral suasion" on its side, as one envious public interest
advocate for a less clearly blessed progressive cause put it

A deservedly despised adversary, "Joe Camel" and his progenitors in the
tobacco industry, as its foil

It also had a board of directors that was uncommonly willing to fight. As
Schneider says: "Our coalition board really took a major risk in seeking out
Vinny and moving on an aggressive electoral approach. That was very much
out of our group's comfort level. It was not something we had ever done." The
fact that the board was willing to risk it all to achieve this tax and hopefully
grow stronger shows the Rabid Third nature of the group. By contrast, when
DeMarco set out to persuade other state tobacco control coalitions to engage
in the election process, they shied away.

Question 7. Filling Gaps: What Do We Need to Develop?

Eric Gally, Kari Appler, and Glenn Schneider, the key staff members of the Smoke Free Maryland Coalition, took stock in 1997 and began
to view Vincent DeMarco as the missing resource in their failed campaigns
to persuade the Maryland legislature to raise the cigarette tax. Gally recognized DeMarco as "the master of the rest of Maryland." What exactly did that
mean?

What could DeMarco add to the Smoke Free Maryland effort? Certainly,
he brought a different kind and quality of campaign leadership, which
I examine in the next chapter. He also brought an aggregation of critical
resources that the Smoke Free Maryland Coalition lacked, including the
following:

Potential new allies among the more than 150 faith, labor, education, and
civic groups and other recruits to his gun control campaigns whose trust
he had earned

Progressive funding sources not shy of funding advocacy, who had learned
that he delivered what he promised—all too rare in philanthropy—which
gave them confidence in his next undertaking

Good relations with Maryland's governor, who had become frustrated in 1997 with what he viewed as the Smoke Free Maryland Coalition's inflexibility; with the attorney general; and with a fair number of legislators with whom he had worked closely on gun control

Journalists and editors—political, as well as health—who had also come to know, trust, and like him and for whom his earlier successes provided exactly the kind of credibility he needed for his next undertaking (The coalition staff had developed some of these relationships, but they lacked the strategy of integrating media advocacy as a primary tool in its campaigns.)

Networks of community activists in every corner of the state whom he had led in the gun control battles

His brain trust and key strategists, especially lobbyist Len Lucchi and media maven Bernie Horn

The wise counsel and emotional ballast of that equally experienced organizer, his wife, Molly Mitchell

Perhaps most important, a strategic perspective gained from his six gun control campaigns that was free of the constraints that experienced tobacco control advocates imposed on themselves by clinging to their customary way of campaigning

After taking stock of the advocacy resources they had, the Smoke Free Maryland leaders knew what they needed: Vincent DeMarco, with all the resources he brought with him. As DeMarco, in turn, assessed the needs of the cigarette tax campaign and saw what gaps remained to be filled, he drew upon his gun control advocacy experience to lay out an expensive and varied set of needs, and then proceeded to meet them:

1. *Money.* Overcoming the Smoke Free Maryland Board's incredulity at the vast sums of both philanthropic and non-tax-deductible money DeMarco told them they would need, he raised both.

2. *Polls.* DeMarco needed expensive polls for multiple strategic purposes, not least to shape the campaign and to provide credibility to the media and potential partners.

3. *An independent campaign organization.* He needed an organization that could focus all its energies on the 1997–1999 tax campaign, without holding back for fear of jeopardizing competing organizational objectives; an organization with managerial authority and flexibility; a new umbrella for a much larger coalition; and a new name that brought a new identity—the Maryland Children's Initiative.

4. *A vastly expanded coalition.* Under the MCI umbrella, DeMarco needed

to gather broad faith, education, youth advocacy, and civic leadership that would signify the shift in frame from taxation and tobacco control to youth welfare.

5. *Authoritative voices.* A special need was authoritative testimony on the benefits to the poor of higher cigarette taxes, which was developed through Bishop Miles and other clergy with poor congregants.

6. *Momentum.* The new campaign needed to develop the image of an operation gaining momentum to grab and hold the attention of the media and, hence, to gain credibility in Annapolis.

7. *Elections.* To make and hold power holders accountable, primary and general election campaigns were needed before a serious effort could be made to seek action from the legislature.

When Baltimore health commissioner Peter Beilenson later recruited DeMarco to lead a universal health-care campaign for Maryland, he, too, acquired the cumulative networks of organizations, political and community leaders, journalists, and funding sources that DeMarco had cultivated. Ten years later, DeMarco's TFK colleagues were able to call upon his exponentially expanding network of national faith leaders.

In taking on the far more politically and economically complex issues involved in attaining health care for all Marylanders, DeMarco was fully capable of organizing the stakeholder and town hall meetings—as well as the polling—that the coalition needed to discover what was politically attainable in the foreseeable future. The campaign also needed the Johns Hopkins health-care experts and the Lewin Group's economic experts to design a feasible health care for all plan, as well as to provide the power of respected authority behind it.

Technical Assistance

In an ideal advocacy world, state or local advocates would know exactly what they need in terms of technical support, or whether they need any help at all. In this world, they often know they need money but don't think they need advocacy training, media advocacy help, or strategic planning guidance. Indeed, they often resent "outside experts."

Progressive foundations and national advocacy organizations like The Robert Wood Johnson Foundation and TFK have long thought they ought to provide technical assistance to their grantees or local chapters to help them achieve their goals. But few foundation program officers have had enough grassroots advocacy experience even to evaluate the proposals of aspiring technical assistance providers. Too often, then, foundations force upon their grantees the *least* useful forms of technical assistance, while their grantees don't know to ask for what might be the *most* useful forms.

Thus Karla Sneegas, the politically insightful director of Indiana's tobacco control program, with no functioning advocacy coalition in place, sought help from TFK. As canny an advocate as she was, Sneegas still did not know exactly what form that help should take. For their part, DeMarco and his TFK colleagues did not at the outset envision as their greatest contribution to state advocacy the creation of a *national* faith network that could in turn activate state faith tobacco control advocacy.

The outline of the DeMarco/TFK alliance in support of state tobacco control in Part III reflects a useful model for technical assistance. After a discouraging start, DeMarco and TFK's Peter Fisher and Patricia Sosa recognized that building Faith United Against Tobacco was the best route for recruiting state faith leaders to the tobacco and health cause. The Robert Wood Johnson Foundation program officers supporting TFK's work did not dictate what to provide the states. To find out what would help most, TFK put experienced advocacy organizers in the field, working hand in hand with state advocates—for example, placing Aaron Doeppers in the Midwest, where he bonded with Sneegas in Indiana.

Jointly, with DeMarco and TFK's D.C.-based team, they identified the kinds of assistance that would be both welcome and useful in Indiana. They provided money and staff support for that assistance. Out of this close collaboration arose the Hoosier Faith and Health Coalition. Neither the support staff nor the coalition dictated to the other. The TFK team members did not behave like saviors from Washington, D.C. "Vinny never presented himself as an outsider," Sneegas says. "He is as much a part of this coalition as anyone else. If you ask the people on the coalition, they would identify him as a member of the coalition—not as some high-paid consultant that's flown in. 'Consultant' would never be a word, ever, ever, ever, that would be associated with Vinny's name."

Question 8. First Steps: How Do We Begin?

How do we begin to build now toward ultimate legislative action? What are the most effective first steps we can take? Perhaps the most important innovation that DeMarco introduced in his campaign strategies was the action he did *not* take first—lobbying the legislature. He deliberately stayed away from legislators for up to two years, in some cases to their annoyance. We can summarize the first steps in DeMarco's campaigns, based on his strategic plans: get the money, take the poll, determine the precise objective, organize and name the campaign organization, build the coalition through a resolution-signature campaign, launch the coalition, and initiate statewide public education. No direct lobbying, yet. The health-care campaign, for instance, needed more than two years just to develop the plan.

Question 9. Strategic Flexibility: What Do We Do When the Plan Isn't Working, Runs into Unforeseen Roadblocks, or Confronts Unanticipated Opportunities?

As they would for any long journey, campaign organizers need to check their course at every stage. They need to reevaluate strategy needs, revisiting each of the preceding eight questions (Are we aiming at the right audiences? Are we reaching them? and so on).

DeMarco would develop in each campaign a discrete plan for their beginning, middle, end, and even aftermath. Even so, he remains acutely attuned to the political environment affecting the course of a campaign and is ready to make minor tactical shifts and even radical course corrections when they are needed. An example of a minor tactical shift: the first public action in the MCI campaign was the trumpeted release to the media of the first campaign poll findings. The result: virtually no media traction. DeMarco regrouped. Several weeks later, with a new cast of sponsoring organizations, he released the results again. This time the news gained the desired headlines.

A major painful shift came in 1998 during the same campaign. To win the essential active support for the cigarette tax increase of Senate Budget and Taxation Committee chair Barbara Hoffman, DeMarco had to strike from the bill the allocations of the proceeds painstakingly negotiated to strengthen the incentives of his core partners. The real pain came when one group waged guerilla warfare against the change, breaching the unified campaign support, though the steadfastness of the other partners sustained the momentum of the tobacco tax.

Following a coherent plan is one rule. A usually overriding rule is following your inside leader or leaders. Governor Glendening was the campaign's powerful and committed leader for the 1999 tax increase. Without his leadership, the increase would be effectively killed, especially in the Senate, where Glendening would have to go toe-to-toe with Senate President Miller. Though the governor had signed the MCI pledge to seek a tax increase of $1.50, when he chose to seek a $1.00 increase instead, DeMarco quietly shifted again. MCI backed the $1.00 increase.

Unlike that 1997–1999 campaign, the Health Care for All! effort that evolved between 2000 and 2007 continuously shape-shifted in response to a series of unanticipated disasters and several opportunities. As early as the end of 2000, the campaign had to relinquish the organizers' vision of fundamental systemic change from an insurer-dominated to a single-payer health-care system. The polls, the stakeholder meetings, and the public town meetings around the state led DeMarco and Baltimore health commissioner Peter Beilenson to conclude that they could hope to bring health care to all Marylanders only by reforming, not replacing, the current system.

Among the campaigns we have examined, it was in this Health Care for All! effort that the single largest monkey wrench in DeMarco's well-laid plans landed: the defeat of Lieutenant Governor Kathleen Kennedy Townsend in the 2002 gubernatorial race. Virtually every political prognosticator had labeled Townsend a near-certain winner. DeMarco had developed a plan that dedicated the years 2000 to 2002 to public education and to building a coalition of more than two thousand members ready to form behind Townsend, a close DeMarco ally, in the governor's office. With the November 2002 elections, he confronted instead a Republican governor, Robert Ehrlich, a determined foe of any such health-care expansion.

Nonetheless, DeMarco came up with a series of interim, incremental, and positive steps toward the Health Care for All! goals that politically circumvented the governor's power yet kept the coalition energized. On the Fair Share provision of the bill, in particular, the powerful business community was either split for and against or—the largest segment—was neutral. DeMarco sensed that the Democratic leadership of both the state House and Senate—not least his sometime hair shirt, Senate President Miller—were looking for a politically potent issue with which to confront the governor. While continuing to call for enactment of the overall Health Care for All! bill, DeMarco seized this opportunity to change course once again and focus all the coalition's resources and energy first on enacting the bill, and then on successfully overriding the governor's veto.

In 2006, DeMarco began to visualize an opportunity in the fall election, when it looked possible that a progressive Democrat would replace Ehrlich. He did not believe that the full Health Care for All! bill was achievable yet, even with a supportive governor, but he saw a chance to enact another element of the overall plan: an increase in the cigarette tax to fund the expansion of Medicaid coverage to Maryland adults living just above the poverty line. Once again, DeMarco departed from an element of the original plan—a thirty-six-cent increase, bringing the full tax to one dollar—this time to strengthen it. He thought a thirty-six-cent increase would not be a sufficiently strong cause to energize the coalition, so he decided on a full dollar increase.

As the legislature convened for the 2007 Special Session, DeMarco painfully reversed course again, persuading his core partners to agree to separate the cigarette tax increase from the Medicaid expansion to satisfy the political (and ego) needs of both the governor and the Senate president; he knew that the committed House speaker would continue the fight to fund Medicaid expansion. Despite grumbling among his allies, DeMarco kept the coalition intact. In early 2008, when the budget crunch came, Speaker Mike Busch and his House lieutenants protected the Medicaid funding. DeMarco's flexibility had proved the right move, but he had taken a real risk, forced upon him by the shifting sands of the political landscape.

15

A Fistful of Campaign Leadership Roles

"There are some people who are natural leaders," says TFK president Matt Myers, "but it would be a mistake to suggest that it requires a unique person to do many of the things that Vinny does." You certainly don't have to be Vinny DeMarco to adopt the generic strategic and tactical lessons I've extracted so far from the case stories. Now, I examine lessons in the leadership roles that mark a successful campaign. This is a trickier task. Not everyone can take on DeMarco's unique set of leadership traits and skills. (Nor does every campaign leader need to rise at five o'clock every morning to go running in the park belting out Neapolitan songs.) Yet it is possible for any campaign organizer, or aspiring organizer, to be cognizant of the full complement of leadership tools and traits that—*combined in the collective leadership* of a policy advocacy campaign—can enhance the probability of success. If I am that organizer, it is incumbent upon me first to examine dispassionately the roles I am capable of performing myself. Then I am in a position to identify or recruit to the campaign team members who can fill the leadership gaps.

For more than twenty years, my colleagues and I at the Advocacy Institute in Washington, D.C., especially my co-directors David Cohen and Kathleen Sheekey, extracted from our own experience and the study of others' efforts some useful empirical insights about the leadership of successful policy advocacy campaigns. We gradually developed and named a set of needed leadership roles, which we call the Leadership Taxonomy:

1. Strategist
2. Organizer/campaign builder
3. Strategic communicator
4. Visionary
5. Insider advocate

6. Fund-raiser
7. Statesperson
8. Policy expert

(To clear up possible confusion over "insider advocate" and "inside advocate": I have focused abundant attention in this book on the critical role played by inside advocates—power holders such as governors and legislative leaders. The taxonomy does not include this role, since inside leaders largely function independently of the advocacy organization.)

Several caveats: First, each role is obviously idealized—no person or collection of people can ever be quite this good (or saintly). Second, there are good reasons why we keep tinkering with the categories—they are slippery; they overlap; all are not always necessary for a successful campaign. For example, if the main advocates for the policy in question happen to be fearsome inside leaders, such as the governor, House leader, and Senate president, little outside leadership may be needed at all.

DeMarco as Exemplary Campaign Leader

Vincent DeMarco comes as close as anyone I've known or studied to fully occupying several of these leadership roles. He fits, most obviously, the descriptions that follow of strategist, strategic communicator, fund-raiser, and organizer/campaign builder. He is an especially good fit, I confess, because I've modified and expanded some of the taxonomy categories and descriptions to reflect the leadership lessons that emerge from observing his campaigns for this book. He also partly fills the roles of visionary and insider. Finally, he is neither statesman nor policy expert, but as organizer he finds leaders already inside the coalition or recruits new leaders who fit these roles.

There are naysayers to my assessment of DeMarco, fiercest among them his formidable opponent in several campaigns, lobbyist Bruce Bereano. Though Bereano understood that I considered DeMarco an exemplary campaigner, he did not temper his disagreement: "I am not, and I never have been, a Vinny DeMarco fan." The kind of issues DeMarco won, says Bereano, are a cinch for any lobbyist. "Not only are the issues DeMarco chooses any lobbyist's dream," Bereano adds, but

> some of the battles that have been won, he has not really won them. It has been the political leaders. For example, there were two times where there was a substantial increase in the tobacco tax—okay. But in both instances, the proposal was dead in the water until there came a time where the governor

stepped in aggressively, or the Senate president or the speaker stepped in. Vinny was able to stand up there and spin it and say, "I won." Had the governor or had the presiding officers not entered the fray, the proposal would have gone nowhere.

Bereano has some of the facts right, but his accounts of these legislative events omit crucial elements. Yes, DeMarco chooses popular issues, as evidenced by polls that show not just citizen support, but support strong enough to move significant numbers of votes in elections, depending on the positions candidates take on that issue. Yet, as Bereano acknowledges, legislative action on these issues was "dead in the water" before DeMarco began to organize massive citizen political power behind them. DeMarco ally Congressman Chris Van Hollen (who, as a state senator in Maryland, led several DeMarco-inspired legislative campaigns) adds what Bereano left out, what galvanizes inside leaders into action: "Vinny makes it clear that there is this whole grassroots army of people who are paying attention—and who will hold people accountable at the ballot box." Similarly, Bereano is right when he argues that DeMarco's successes were achieved only because the governor and key legislative leaders supported the issues, but he again leaves out the critical element: how DeMarco gained that leadership's support. For example, although Governor Glendening strongly believed in tobacco control and in principle supported a cigarette tax increase, he was reluctant to use his depleted political capital to fight for one. Only when DeMarco had mobilized a sea of voters behind the increase and put pressure on the governor and his rivals to sign the pledge, and only after DeMarco had successfully made the pledge a winning issue for Glendening, did the governor commit wholeheartedly to the fight. In the Fair Share health-care bill, DeMarco designed the legislation to give the Senate president, a strong partisan Democrat, an issue with which to bludgeon the Republican governor. In the cigarette tax/Medicaid expansion success in the 2007 Special Session, the governor and legislative leadership support was a direct result of a DeMarco strategy: the media advocacy campaign that elevated health-care expansion to the top of the voters' priority list—making it impossible for the leadership to ignore.

Leadership Taxonomy Roles That DeMarco Fills

1. Strategist

Strategy planning is part of every campaign organizer's toolkit. DeMarco's version is unusual in two ways. First, instead of drawing upon strategies handed down by other campaigners, DeMarco has developed a campaign template drawn almost entirely from his own trial and error in the course of more than a dozen discrete campaigns over twenty years. Second, instead of the piecemeal design typical of issue campaigns—an organizing component, a lobbying component, a communications component, and so on—DeMarco's plans seamlessly integrate the components into the whole. As Bernie Horn observes: "Too many advocates learn the craft of particular pieces of a campaign: how to put on a conference; how to do a TV ad; how to do a TV campaign. This they learn over time. And so their idea of good advocacy is doing the thing that they've learned very well."

"Vinny has perfected the ultimate formula for building progressive coalitions and advancing the progressive agenda," says Len Lucchi. "It's hard work, but it's also very simple." What Lucchi calls "a gross simplification" of what DeMarco does still captures its essence: "He takes a problem, defines the problem, gets those who have power to commit to collusion. He runs a campaign to educate the voting public about it. Hopefully, he elects supportive legislative candidates in the process. Then, just as important, he holds the people who pledge in the campaign to do the right thing to keep that pledge. It's a brilliant way to do it."

As a strategist, DeMarco is for the most part soberly rational; each campaign plan is firmly grounded in the experience of earlier campaigns. His colleague Horn insists, however, that "while Vinny's a great strategist, sometimes he doesn't know why he's doing what he's doing." Glenn Schneider tempers this observation: "Though Vinny is highly intuitive and usually right on, he won't let that stand in the way of doing something that he feels is anti-intuitive if strong advice steers him elsewhere." For example, Schneider says, DeMarco did not want to introduce the Health Care for All! bill before the Fair Share battle. Staff convinced him that this would be out of step with what the coalition wanted, Schneider says, an opinion confirmed by "key informant group interviews." DeMarco gave in, "and we introduced the full bill."

DeMarco laughed when I asked him about his intuition. What came to mind was his decision in 2006, when the Republican governor stood in the way of advancing the grander health care for all plan, to recommend seeking the one-dollar cigarette tax increase to fund Medicaid expansion, which veered from that plan. "I just had a feeling that we needed to do something different than what we were doing. We had to go for the dollar tobacco tax for health care. It just was a deep instinctive feeling for me that that was the way. Sometimes I see a road ahead—we all have that—without analyzing it through. There's an instinctive feeling that when the road is blocked for now, we have to go this other way."

Because DeMarco's "instinctive feeling" is grounded in years of experience, let's call this informed intuition.

2. Organizer/Campaign Builder

Organizer/campaign builders sustain coalitions. They create space for tapping the knowledge gained through their own experience and the experience of others, and initiate new approaches to participation so that diverse voices are heard and their demands heeded. They circumvent organizational turf hurdles; they convene and facilitate, seek to explore differences through civil discourse and debate, and eschew rancorous division. They pay attention to sustaining relationships with colleagues or key allies even when not calling upon them to do something. Builders also heal. Within the campaign, they communicate, communicate, communicate.

DeMarco's "greatest strength," in his wife Molly Mitchell's words, "is how he manages to bring in so many disparate groups and orchestrate them to accomplish so much together." In the same vein, Karla Sneegas, herself a much admired tobacco control organizer/leader in Indiana, says she learned from DeMarco "not to be afraid to bring together what might be considered opposing forces: to bring the conservative Southern Baptists together at the same table where Islam is sitting there and the Catholics and the Jewish community." In her experience, "Vinny's a bridge builder. Our health folks don't really understand how to build bridges. A lot of tobacco control people have been afraid to push our comfort zone by dealing with people who aren't like us. He taught us not to be afraid to put some really different people at the same table." TFK colleague Patricia Sosa insists that DeMarco creates "coalitions that are real. There are a lot of people that are able to put together coalitions that are very impressive—on paper. Vinny creates coalitions with a backbone."

IT'S THE RELATIONSHIPS

Glenn Schneider reflects thoughtfully on the critical role that relationship building plays in the organizing of DeMarco and his team:

> To be a successful organizer, you must understand and embrace two key concepts: satisfying self-interests and forming strong relationships. Why do you do anything in your life? Either you *must* do it (it satisfies an essential need), you *want* to do it (it satisfies a perceived desire), *or* someone you care about asks you to do it (it is part of being in relationship). When recruiting coalition members, think first about recruiting groups that have the most to gain should you win your campaign. With the Fair Share campaign, surely the food service unions and Giant Food, one of Wal-Mart's biggest competitors, had something to gain. But when trying to build broader business support for Fair Share health care, did Vinny start off cold calling? No, he called his neighbors and friends and friends of friends, some of whom owned or operated businesses, and asked them to support the campaign. When they

agreed to endorse, he asked for their help in framing his messages to the business community and later asked them to serve as spokespeople. All of this was possible because a good relationship got his foot in the door.

When Vinny and Co. were trying to build our Health Care for All! Coalition, who did we turn to first? Sure, we thought about those groups who cared about health-care reform. But we also turned to those people and groups with which we had already formed a relationship. Vinny turned to his gun control friends, Rosanna [Miles] to her faith community friends, and I turned to my tobacco control friends. You might not get your friends to support what you are doing, but you will surely get them to listen. Even if they don't endorse your campaign, they may give you hints on how to better approach similar people or groups. They might help you better frame your arguments. Vinny's success is mainly related to his ability to build strong relationships, whether they be with individuals, groups of people, and/or lawmakers. Further, he's not afraid to draw on these relationships for help.

If you want to be a good organizer and advocate, listen carefully for a person or group's self-interest and try to meet it, form strong, trusting, honest, two-way relationships with people, and don't be afraid to ask for help from those "close to home."

NEVER TAKES NO FOR AN ANSWER?
Patricia Sosa says of DeMarco: "Once he gets ahold of you, if you say no, it's no. You have to give him an answer, but once you give him an answer, he respects the answer. But what entices people is that he gives them options. 'Can you do this?' 'No.' 'But can you do this?' Eventually, people feel like, 'Well, I have to do *something*. He's given me ten choices of what I have to do, there's something I'm going to be able to do to contribute.' "

Barrett Duke, chief legislative advocate for the Southern Baptists, echoes Sosa:

> One of the things I always say is that Vinny knows how to take no for an answer. When you tell him no, he leaves it alone. He may come back to you many times for different things, but when you tell him no on one thing, he doesn't come back asking for that again. So he's very respectful of boundaries and what the various groups, individuals, are able to do. It's really been encouraging to a lot of our folks too when they've worked with him, because they found him to be respectful as well. He does not force himself on people. He takes what you give him and he doesn't ask for more.

Duke made this point about DeMarco on a panel discussion with one of DeMarco's oldest and closest colleagues, Bishop Miles. Miles erupted, to the accompaniment of knowing laughter, "Barrett, Vinny never takes no for an answer!"

The truth lies delicately in between.

FOLLOW-UP AND HELP

Another manifestation of DeMarco's persistence—and effectiveness—as an organizer and campaign builder is his virtually instantaneous follow-up to make certain that once a colleague agrees to do something, he or she *does* it, not tomorrow but today. But this follow-up is leavened by DeMarco's readiness to make the task as burden free as possible. Patricia Sosa elaborates:

> Once they say, "Yes, I want to do it," the follow-up is so impeccable that people feel really rewarded. They get excited because they're part of something. Although I have to say that we tease a lot about Vinny the "noodge extraordinaire." But serious work happens. There's a core group of lobbyists in the national headquarters of the denominations that make up Faith United. When there's a project planned, Vinny will send a note to the lobbyists saying: "Project in Richmond, Virginia. We need your people." And everybody sends Vinny names, because they know Vinny will follow up.
>
> Remember, you're a busy person trying to think what to work on next. Then you find these people that are going to help you and facilitate your work and will guide you in a way that works for you. This is a win-win. Vinny keeps taking them to these places where they can make a difference. That's why they love coming back. That's the reason why the follow-up is so key. I would say of all the assets that he brings to the table, his discipline on the follow-up is very key—because it reinforces. You do something, he will reply. He will do exactly what he said he was going to do. That's really valuable.

SUSTAINABILITY

Is DeMarco so overwhelming an organizer/leader that when he leaves, things fall apart? The best organizers leave behind strong organizations with strong leadership. Does DeMarco? No, and yes. After he left Marylanders Against Handgun Abuse, the organization went into slow decline and has never been a significant force since. But Smoke Free Maryland flourished, continuing to gain significant tobacco control achievements to this day. DeMarco constantly put other leaders forward in his media advocacy efforts, leaving himself, as columnist Fraser Smith calls him, "a second paragraph guy." In his health-care advocacy, he has promoted the leadership of both old and new coalition leaders, such as the AARP's chief operating officer. DeMarco's efforts to cultivate leadership beyond himself is manifest: from underpinning the leaders of the national Faith United Against Tobacco, such as United Methodist Jim Winkler and Southern Baptist Richard Land, to the painstaking elevation of the Indiana faith and health coalition. Leadership development was at the forefront, successfully, of his activities.

3. Strategic Communicator

A strategic communicator also spends time and effort cultivating the comfort and trust of key journalists and producers when there is no story to push, so that when the time comes for a story on a matter of concern, the writer or producer is primed not only to respond to campaign press releases, but also to reach out to the strategic communicator in advance for guidance on any related story. DeMarco's media advocacy strategies, and his own role in those strategies, have been so central an element throughout this book that they need no embellishment here.

Leadership Taxonomy Roles That DeMarco Shares

4. Visionary

Is DeMarco a "visionary"? Not as we normally understand the term. Baltimore health commissioner Peter Beilenson fits the bill better in his ongoing espousal of the radical restructuring of Maryland's health care to a single-payer system. Though he understood and concurred in DeMarco's evolving strategies, Beilenson never abandoned that vision. DeMarco, by contrast, focused more on what was politically attainable in the near future. He set aside the single-payer goal when confronted with insurmountable political hurdles—a pragmatic Don Quixote.

Yet in each of his campaigns DeMarco does entertain a vision of the possible that others label a fantasy. This was true of one of his earliest ventures, when he proposed a bill to ban Saturday-night-special handguns. His Young Democrats colleague Bernie Horn told him he was "crazy": "Nobody had passed any gun control legislation on the state or federal level for a decade. Deep into the Reagan years, it was perceived [to be] politically impossible. Yet, with the rest of us dragging our feet, he pulled us into this effort. Passing this bill was a miracle."

We've seen Glenn Schneider convinced that DeMarco had taken leave of his senses when he told the Smoke Free Maryland Board that he could raise unheard-of levels of political funding to fuel a cigarette tax campaign. But he raised the money. When DeMarco took on the leadership of the campaign to achieve health care for all Marylanders, Horn—the consummate pragmatist—was again skeptical: "I thought it was politically impossible, that he was biting off more than he could chew. But he had vision."

Not uncommonly in the campaigns we've observed, DeMarco sees that what others think is impossible can be done. Perhaps not "visionary," but "rational optimist" best captures this quality—no small virtue in a campaigner facing repeated barriers.

5. Insider Advocate

Is DeMarco an influential insider? Throughout this book, I've drawn sharp distinctions between him and Bruce Bereano, whom Senate President Miller called, even after Bereano's conviction for campaign-financing abuse, "one of my closest friends." When Miller first met DeMarco, his opening salvo was, "Oh, you're that bomb-thrower." In contrast, even Bereano respects Len Lucchi as a fellow insider: "I know Len well. I've known him for a long time. He's a down-to-earth, legitimate, friendly guy.... He's honest, he's trustworthy, he's not about himself, he's a team player." What about DeMarco? "None of it," says Bereano, "is Vinny DeMarco." As Lucchi admits, when legislators see DeMarco coming, they sometimes run in the opposite direction: "All of a sudden, the whole hallway clears out; they all run in and hide in their offices."

Among other lobbyists who have worked as allies with DeMarco, however, he has elicited growing respect. "I've been in Annapolis representing Giant on issues since 1973," says Barry Scher. "Four or five years ago, I started hearing about this guy named Vinny DeMarco, and what I heard from other lobbyists was, 'He's a kind of off-the-wall guy. He always has a relentless pursuit of whatever he goes after. But he's a little nutty. You don't want to get associated with that guy. He's really strange, he's really weird; looks like he just got out of bed.'" Scher's opinion is that "Vinny's style is still a little rough at the edges, but [he's] not so much of a nut as was depicted by many of my peers." When he worked closely with DeMarco on the Fair Share bill, Scher found that "once you sit down with Vinny DeMarco, you get to understand that he has, indeed, done his homework. He's very good with facts and figures, and his research was really second to none. I remember at that time saying to myself, 'He's really an astute individual.'" According to Scher, DeMarco "has continued to be very professional, and he's gotten more attention from legislators because of his doing his homework on issues."

Part of DeMarco's success as an insider is his occasional unwillingness to confront those who oppose him. While some allies view this reluctance as a weakness, there's method in it—as is true for some of his other apparent idiosyncrasies. Maggie McIntosh, as a legislator, well understands: "He's not confrontational with people that he knows he needs on his side. So he's not going to be confrontational with people like [Maryland Senate President] Mike Miller. That's really because he's focused on how to get the job done, not because he's afraid of confrontation. That's another mistake a lot of people make, though, is they are confrontational with people that they need." He also doesn't take opposition personally, as Methodist policy advocate Sandy Ferguson observes: "He doesn't hold grudges because he's so focused on the issues. He has a passion, and he doesn't deviate from that."

Bishop Miles observes that DeMarco "will try to work around difference; he will try to see how we can work together. But when it comes down to it, he'll confront"—as he did, memorably, when he decided to run the ads in 1999 attacking the Maryland legislators who filibustered final Senate approval of any cigarette tax increase.

Where DeMarco has truly become an insider is with the inside leaders he has worked with. Not drinking buddies. Not "my closest friends." Instead of picking up the tab for lavish lunches and dinners, the only comestible DeMarco ever parts with—and that sparingly—is an honorary jar of his family's homemade tomato sauce. Among these leaders is Maryland House Speaker Mike Busch, who delivered a fierce public scolding to DeMarco when Busch was chairing Maryland's House Economic Matters Committee. Several years later, when Busch had moved up to speaker of the House, he told me that the "vast majority" of lobbyists he associated with in Annapolis represented corporations or a large coalition of private-sector individuals. "Vinny represents a large coalition of the public sector," Busch says, "and you always want to make sure that you're accountable to them. So Vinny has a lot more influence than a guy flying in from North Carolina representing R. J. Reynolds." Busch saw DeMarco's strategy as finding issues important to the many "constituencies out there that have not had a central focal point to articulate their views." Then "he brings a coalition" to Annapolis, where he succeeds with the legislature because "he can identify people in everyone's community that want to see some kind of change in a particular issue he is advocating for. He connects his issue with faces and leaders in the community and the legislator that's making the vote—and the fact is, elected leaders start to listen and pay attention."

Through the course of his campaigns, DeMarco has nourished working relationships with governors, legislative leaders, committee chairs, and other respected progressive legislators. Together with Len Lucchi and others among his close working allies, such as Glenn Schneider, Bernie Horn, and faith leaders like Bishop Miles and Sandy Ferguson, he has forged a formidable network of influence within the power structure in Annapolis. Therefore, he fits, if somewhat awkwardly, in the category of insider advocate, though he still retains many of the qualities—for both good and ill—of the unwashed outsider. Perhaps, if we need a label, we can call DeMarco the *outsiders' insider.*

6. Fund-raiser

DeMarco is an intrepid fund-raiser, based on early and frequent cultivation of and attention to a core group of funders, who in turn signal to others the effectiveness—and safety—of investing in his ventures. Most of the funds for his work come from foundations whom he cultivates assiduously (with assistance from a skilled grant writer on staff, Suzanne Gilbert). To help raise the hard-to-find non-tax-deductible money he needs for his health-care work, he has gone back to an ally from the gun control campaign twenty years earlier, Colleen Martin-Lauer, who had evolved into a leading fund-raising consultant for progressive causes and candidates. And, to help on all this, DeMarco recruited to his health-care board veteran fund-raisers for good causes with their own wide network of funders, particularly his board treasurer, Joel Rabin.

Filling Leadership Taxonomy Gaps

One of the challenges for organizers is to assess objectively, given their own leadership capacities and roles, what the campaign lacks in the leadership arena. Throughout, this book has shown DeMarco's ability to find the key inside leaders with whom to partner, such as statespeople and policy experts.

7. Statesperson

In virtually every campaign he entered, DeMarco looked to prominent statesmen and stateswomen for public leadership: for gun control, Attorneys General Joseph Curran and Steven Sachs; during the 1997–1999 tobacco tax campaign, Governor Glendening; in the early stages of the health-care campaign, Lieutenant Governor Townsend; in later stages of the health-care campaign, House Speaker Busch and then Governor O'Malley. Ironically, though they were prime adversaries in other campaigns, DeMarco embraced Senate President Miller as a leader in the campaign for the Fair Share bill.

In building the countrywide Faith United Against Tobacco coalition, DeMarco happily ceded the national stage to the prominent faith leaders Jim Winkler, general secretary of the General Board of Church and Society of the United Methodist Church; and to Richard Land—famed or infamous, depending on the issue and the audience—president of the Ethics and Religious Liberty Commission of the Southern Baptist Convention, whom *Newsweek* once described as "God's lobbyist."

8. Policy Expert

DeMarco cannot be an expert in the science of all of the issues he has organized around, at least at first, so again, he turns to others as needed. In his
early gun control campaigns, he sought out Stephen Teret, a public health
professor at Johns Hopkins, to rebut the National Rifle Association's pseudo-
scientific defense of guns. He turned to experts from Johns Hopkins and national groups such as Families USA and Community Catalyst to design the
plan for the Health Care for All! campaign, and to economic experts at the
Lewin Group to uphold its financial integrity. For his political forensic polls,
he recruited nationally respected pollsters such as Celinda Lake, Mark Penn,
and Mark Mellman. On the science of tobacco control, he drew upon research
experts at TFK, Danny McGoldrick and Eric Lindblom.

Within his extended advocacy family, DeMarco relies on many for their
specialized expertise and gifts—so many that it would be exhausting to list
them all. But to illustrate, they include Len Lucchi's lobbying expertise, Bernie
Horn's media advocacy professionalism, and lawyer Michael Pretl's nonprofit
tax expertise ("I'm general counsel for Vinny, Inc.," Pretl jokes). Even with his
own organizing expertise, DeMarco recognizes and leans on the organizing
skills of many others, including Rosanna Miles and her organizing strengths
and networks. And from the very beginning of the tobacco tax campaign,
Glenn Schneider has been an indispensable health policy expert, as well as
strategist and implementer. Yet in some areas DeMarco acquires enough expertise to become a substantive and political resource for the media, as Maggie McIntosh testifies: "Now, he is viewed as one of the experts on health care
in the state—a leading expert. He is a go-to person on health care in the state
of Maryland because he has tremendous command of the issue and is very
well respected."

Conclusion: Energy, Exuberance, Authenticity, and Optimism

The impatience, restlessness, relentlessness, pushiness—qualities
that sometimes craze DeMarco's friends and colleagues—reflect the boundless
energy that is so essential to DeMarco's follow-up to every commitment: his
e-mails, calls, smartphone outreach, and touching of every ally, every journalist within reach, everyone whom he has asked or tasked, every bruised ego
needing salve.

DeMarco's exuberance, observes Len Lucchi, who has put up with his
friend's foibles longer than almost anyone else, is "infectious." Johns Hopkins
psychologist Kay Redfield Jamison celebrates the importance to society of

exuberance in her book of the same name. I've known no one who embodies her definition of the term more aptly than DeMarco: "Exuberance is an abounding, ebullient, effervescent emotion. It is kinetic and unrestrained, joyful, irrepressible. . . . Exuberance leaps, bubbles, and overflows, . . . spreads upward and outward like pollen toted by dancing bees, and in this carrying ideas are moved and actions taken."

Among Bruce Bereano's complaints about DeMarco is, "It's all about him." But I think he's dead wrong. Yes, DeMarco takes much joy in his work. Yes, he's happy when the media tells his campaign stories the way he wants them to. But it's not about him, but about the progress of the campaign. Yes, he has a strong ego. A leader needs one, especially in dealing with strong-willed allies like Beilenson and strong-willed sometime opponents like Miller. But none of those who work for DeMarco believe that he is driven by egotism or ego-centricity.

The reflections of Matt Myers, TFK president, complement similar quotations about DeMarco from others throughout this book, among them Bishop Miles's declaration that he has "never met a more authentic person." Myers views DeMarco as both disciplined and focused, "not allowing ego or other distractions to get in the way. Vinny doesn't allow himself to get sidetracked by the issues on which he disagrees with people. He doesn't let that get in the way of his relationship with those people or in his organizing and work with those people. And one of the reasons I think that people trust him is because it's genuine." Myers sees DeMarco as capable of setting sound objective goals, working toward them, and "understanding what it's really all about and not letting ideology, passion, personality, get in the way. In that respect, he's the ultimate problem solver. Frankly, I think it's the best of what American political figures historically have done, and that we don't do so well anymore."

Epilogue

What Would Vinny Do?

In the flush of excitement and optimism that followed the election of Barack Obama in November 2008, I cited the DeMarco factor as a model in a piece I wrote for the December 15 issue of *The Nation* ("Election's Over—Time to Begin"). There, I speculated that the thousands of trained, highly motivated organizers and the millions of volunteers and contributors who made Obama's victory possible could now be mobilized to make certain that his legislative agenda was enacted. Some of that has indeed happened. But it now seems clear that the organizing energy of the electoral campaign has been difficult to recharge even through vigorous online action alerts and petitions, potluck suppers with cell-phone trees, lobbying, letters, and rallies. Much of what Obama has sought—and voters have supported—has been blocked. The Bush regime is gone, but the corrupt power of the moneyed lobbies is not.

When I asked Rosanna Miles what she and others would do when DeMarco was no longer leading them, she replied: "We'd carry on. We'd be sad, but when we were faced with a problem, we'd always ask ourselves, 'What would Vinny do?'" Now, having looked at how DeMarco approaches various political challenges, we can do the same. What might a progressive president's political advisors and advocacy leaders borrow from DeMarco's campaign template to reverse the imbalance of political power between voters and lobbyists in the coming years?

They might learn that transforming unfocused public yearning for systemic change that challenges entrenched power takes long-range planning, exhaustive relationship building, and patience uncharacteristic for Americans—that is, fundamentally, that successful legislative organizing cannot be built during the few months of a legislative or election campaign, but must be built over years.

DeMarco's campaigns demonstrate that organizing the leadership of groups, not just individual voters, is the most effective way of building *sustained* support for legislation. But turning to existing coalitions of customary allies who represent small fractions of the electorate is never sufficient. DeMarco has repeatedly succeeded in assembling groups into fresh alliances, bringing together, for example, the diverse forces of public health advocates and faith groups in faith and health coalitions.

We have seen that such mobilization can be promoted systematically by strategies such as coalition-organizing resolutions, legislative trial runs to ferret out legislative supporters and opponents, primary and general election concrete pledge campaigns—all accompanied by relentless media advocacy and sustained lobbying. What DeMarco and his allies have taught us is that legislative success over economically and politically potent opposition is possible only when elected policymakers understand that the will of the voters for the passage of legislation is broad and deep. That can happen only when there is demonstrable evidence in the form of elections that vindicate support for such legislation and punish those who oppose it. Get concrete, redeemable pledges from candidates before they are elected, and defeat even a handful of candidates who refuse to pledge, and you have erected a bulwark against the otherwise seductive pleading, lubricated by campaign contributions, of insider lobbyists.

In legislative and election campaigns to come, the near paralysis in our current political environment manifestly calls for unorthodox strategies. In searching for effective change, public health and social justice strategists might also well begin by asking first, "What would Vinny do?"

Acknowledgments

So many kind people contributed to this book that I need to begin by grouping them, and then, at hazard, naming those who most compensated for my insufficiencies. Yet, this leaves unacknowledged too many more whose contributions were not small and others whose generosity as interviewees or as previous writers about DeMarco are absent from the book, not because of their lack of added value, but because the sum of all would have sunk the book by their weight.

There are two complementary pillars upon which this book stands, without whom it could not have gone forward: Michael Ames, both publisher and editor at Vanderbilt University Press, and Fred Mann, Joe Marx, and Michael Berman at The Robert Wood Johnson Foundation. Each had faith that the book would be worthwhile before a word had been written; Fred, Joe, and Michael offered encouragement and, through a Foundation grant, covered the expenses of the research and writing. The book took almost a year longer than planned; they never wavered in their support.

Next, there were DeMarco's closest colleagues, whose stories and insights make this book come alive far beyond my own narrative voice. Their interviews were my primary source; their inexhaustible patience in reviewing successive flawed drafts, my safeguard against factual errors, missed insights, and misguided lessons: DeMarco's wife Molly; his allies from Hopkins days, especially Bernie Horn and Len Lucchi; his tobacco tax and health-care campaign teammates, especially Glenn Schneider and Rosanna Miles. Schneider, along with DeMarco, served triple duty: their interviews were the most exhaustive; their stern corrections of factual error, the most exacting; their insights, the most revealing. It is no accident that they are the most quoted. The Campaign for Tobacco-Free Kids team, led by Patricia Sosa, gave unstinting time and effort to get right the remarkable story of Faith United Against Tobacco.

Before I turned to researching this book, journalists Tom Waldron and Catherine Pierre had ably researched and written about DeMarco's ventures.

They both generously shared with me the interviews they had conducted, many of them contemporaneously with the events I have chronicled. I conducted more than fifty more; all together, the total interviews that were the primary source for this book number well over seventy. They range from unabashed admirers (mother Rosa comes first to mind) to unapologetic adversaries, such as tobacco lobbyist Bruce Bereano, who, undaunted by my confessed admiration for DeMarco, nonetheless readily agreed to share his passion to debunk what he views as the DeMarco myth.

There were, at the time of this writing, as I have told, more than eight thousand names in the address book of DeMarco's smartphone. I didn't talk to all of them, but I did talk to a goodly number of friends and allies outside the inner circle; even short conversations with family members and neighbors shed light. To all, I am grateful, including many who are not quoted and whose names are not cited in this book, who nonetheless helped guide me.

My next acknowledgments are tinged with dread for the future. The reporters, columnists, and editorial writers, especially those of the *Baltimore Sun*, who reported and commented on, praised and needled, supported and challenged DeMarco and his campaigns, strung together, would alone have sourced a solid book. As I noted in the introduction, quotations (including the book's title) from the *Sun*'s senior political columnist throughout most of the events that take place in this book, C. Fraser Smith, grace many of these pages. But others covered the DeMarco stories consistently and vigorously. Their bylines, too, are spread throughout. I doubt that we shall see the quantity and quality of such coverage from daily print newspapers ever again.

Finally, there is another category of help that matches all the others—my editors and reviewers: Bobbe Needham, the book's developmental editor, reviewed every draft chapter early and late; then with an uncanny blend of encouraging kindness and keen sensitivity to my prolixity, she set me straight. Now serving as editor, Michael Ames shepherded me firmly throughout, with remedial prescriptions that will remain forever posted on my writing wall. He also chose two uncommonly insightful reviewers, John Atlas and Andrew Mott, who eased my anxieties with kind praise and then delivered shock treatment on the draft manuscript's lacunae. If you ever need transcriptions of arcane subject interviews, find Kay Carlsen, who takes pride in getting every name and obscure reference right. My patient mentor and friend, political scientist Charles Lindblom, from whom I learn at lunch every week, also read each draft and offered broad guidance all the way through (mostly kind but perhaps even more helpful, in one draft section, which has now been drastically revised, he wrote, "I stopped reading this after the first few pages"). Finally, despite all this help, Jessie Dolch, the copy editor, found much too much to cure, and did so with wisdom and tact.

Within our family, my son Mark, now a veteran public health advocate and counselor, read, guided, and encouraged; my stepson Dan, the classicist, provided exquisitely nuanced edits; and my daughter Amy provided informed encouragement just as my spirits flagged. My wife Anna lived with me and the book for three years, a needed source of good sense, emergency doses of kindness, and a constant reminder of all the things other than writing that make my life joyous.

Index